MOTIVATIONAL INTERVIEWING
IN DIABETES CARE

Applications of Motivational Interviewing

Stephen Rollnick, William R. Miller,
and Theresa B. Moyers, Series Editors

www.guilford.com/AMI

Since the publication of Miller and Rollnick's classic *Motivational Interviewing*, now in its third edition, MI has been widely adopted as a tool for facilitating change. This highly practical series includes general MI resources as well as books on specific clinical contexts, problems, and populations. Each volume presents powerful MI strategies that are grounded in research and illustrated with concrete "how-to-do-it" examples.

**Motivational Interviewing in Health Care:
Helping Patients Change Behavior**
*Stephen Rollnick, William R. Miller,
and Christopher C. Butler*

**Building Motivational Interviewing Skills:
A Practitioner Workbook**
David B. Rosengren

Motivational Interviewing with Adolescents and Young Adults
Sylvie Naar-King and Mariann Suarez

Motivational Interviewing in Social Work Practice
Melinda Hohman

Motivational Interviewing in the Treatment of Anxiety
Henny A. Westra

**Motivational Interviewing, Third Edition:
Helping People Change**
William R. Miller and Stephen Rollnick

Motivational Interviewing in Groups
Christopher C. Wagner and Karen S. Ingersoll, with Contributors

**Motivational Interviewing in the Treatment
of Psychological Problems, Second Edition**
Hal Arkowitz, William R. Miller, and Stephen Rollnick, Editors

Motivational Interviewing in Diabetes Care
Marc P. Steinberg and William R. Miller

MOTIVATIONAL INTERVIEWING IN DIABETES CARE

Marc P. Steinberg
William R. Miller

THE GUILFORD PRESS
New York   London

© 2015 The Guilford Press
A Division of Guilford Publications, Inc.
370 Seventh Avenue, Suite 1200, New York, NY 10001
www.guilford.com

Printed in the United States of America

This book is printed on acid-free paper.

Last digit is print number: 9 8 7 6 5 4

The authors have checked with sources believed to be reliable in their efforts to
provide information that is complete and generally in accord with the standards
of practice that are accepted at the time of publication. However, in view of the
possibility of human error or changes in behavioral, mental health, or medical
sciences, neither the authors, nor the editor and publisher, nor any other party
who has been involved in the preparation or publication of this work warrants
that the information contained herein is in every respect accurate or complete, and
they are not responsible for any errors or omissions or the results obtained from
the use of such information. Readers are encouraged to confirm the information
contained in this book with other sources.

Library of Congress Cataloging-in-Publication Data

Steinberg, Marc P.
  Motivational interviewing in diabetes care / Marc P. Steinberg, William R. Miller.
     pages cm. — (Applications of motivational interviewing)
  Includes bibliographical references and index.
  ISBN 978-1-4625-2163-0 (paperback) — ISBN 978-1-4625-2155-5 (hardcover)
  1. Diabetes—Treatment.   2. Motivational interviewing.   I. Miller, William R.,
  1944– II. Title.
  RC660.S72 2015
  616.4′620651—dc23
                                                          2015018263

*To my family—Deb, Peter, and Claire—
for the light you bring to my life*
—MPS

*For my sister Frances, who died at age 8
from complications of diabetes*
—WRM

About the Authors

Marc P. Steinberg, MD, FAAP, developed a focus on diabetes care during his 32 years of practice as a physician. He became increasingly interested in working more effectively with people struggling with or disengaged in the self-care of chronic conditions, and, since ending his medical practice in 2013, has focused on training health care providers in motivational interviewing. Dr. Steinberg has written articles on motivational interviewing in *Diabetes Spectrum* and is a member of the Motivational Interviewing Network of Trainers. He belongs to the national medical honor society Alpha Omega Alpha and is a Fellow of the American Academy of Pediatrics. He has maintained an active lifestyle with type 1 diabetes for more than 40 years.

William R. Miller, PhD, is Emeritus Distinguished Professor of Psychology and Psychiatry at the University of New Mexico. Particularly interested in the psychology of change, he introduced the concept of motivational interviewing in 1983. Dr. Miller has published over 400 professional articles and chapters and 50 books, including *Motivational Interviewing*, now in its third edition, and *Motivational Interviewing in Health Care*. He is a recipient of the international Jellinek Memorial Award, two career achievement awards from the American Psychological Association, and an Innovators in Combating Substance Abuse Award from the Robert Wood Johnson Foundation, as well as many other honors. The Institute for Scientific Information has listed him as one of the world's most highly cited researchers.

Preface

Health care is simple: just tell people what to do!

Work would be a lot easier and we could all get home at a more reasonable hour if treating people with diabetes consisted of just giving them a list of what to do as they departed happily, bound on a journey toward better health. Our work is challenging precisely because our patients' health outcomes do not rely only on what we do. How people manage their diabetes (or don't) after they leave our offices—how they live their lives—will probably have bigger impact than most of what we do in our offices. People with diabetes often find treatment difficult because it disrupts their long-standing habits and violates the comforts of the status quo. Furthermore, the progressive nature of diabetes often necessitates adjustments in treatment and self-care routines, so that change becomes an ongoing issue in diabetes care.

This book offers what we hope will be a refreshing perspective for reframing diabetes care, namely, using motivational interviewing (MI) in discussions about change. MI uses evidence-based counseling skills for helping people change their own health behavior. Instead of merely telling patients what to do, MI offers a particular way of listening to evoke their own ideas about and solutions for the challenges they face in taking care of their diabetes.

Have you ever looked over the daily list of people who are coming to see you and experienced dread because a "difficult person" was on the list, someone who requires lots of your energy or evokes feelings of frustration or hopelessness? We hope that this book will offer you a pleasantly different way to approach and experience your work in diabetes health care, one that may be particularly helpful with more "difficult" patients.

MI can be particularly useful when time is short. There is a natural tendency to think, "I don't have much time so I just have to tell them what to do," and you can then record in your notes that you did in fact tell them. However, for reasons explored in the early chapters of this book, telling people what to do is usually not very effective in changing their behavior, and frequently it can even backfire. When you don't have much time and what you hope for is behavior change on the part of your patient, MI is a good way to use the time you have.

Part I offers a succinct overview of MI—what it is, how it works, and some basics that you need to know to get started practicing it. Part II, which constitutes the largest portion of the book, illustrates the use of MI in common everyday challenges that are a part of professional diabetes care, such as:

- Newly diagnosed diabetes
- Needed lifestyle changes
- Using medications
- Introducing insulin use to a person with type 2 diabetes
- Conversations with parents and adolescents who have type 1 diabetes
- Talking to concerned family members
- What to say during follow-up visits to encourage continued health behavior change
- Managing complications of diabetes
- Alcohol/drug use as a complicating factor
- Psychological stress and depression as issues in diabetes management

The final section, Part III, addresses three related topics:

- How to learn and improve your skills in MI
- Using MI in group visits
- MI as a tool in diabetes prevention and the worldwide epidemic of type 2 diabetes

Taken together, these chapters introduce you to the spirit and practice of this well-developed and tested method for having conversations with patients about change. We offer you some practical tools that you can try right away, though it does take some time to develop your skills in this clinical style. We hope that at least we can give you a taste of this approach and the opportunity to see how differently patients can respond. It might even whet your appetite for some additional training and coaching to sharpen your MI skills, which can be so useful in health care more generally. May it also make your own work feel lighter, more enjoyable and rewarding, and more effective in helping your patients with diabetes.

Contents

PART I

MOTIVATIONAL INTERVIEWING AS A CLINICAL STYLE

CHAPTER 1

Why Don't People Do What We Tell Them to Do?

Diabetes involves challenging work for both caregivers and patients. Few conditions are associated with such a complex array of lifestyle and medical treatment issues. The health consequences of uncontrolled diabetes are both serious and preventable (Diabetes Control and Complications Trial Research Group, 1993; UKPDS Study Group, 1998), and there are clear metrics and target values for quality diabetes care (hemoglobin A1C, low-density lipoprotein [LDL] cholesterol, and blood pressure). Yet, despite best efforts, the majority of diabetes patients (49–99%) in both developed and underdeveloped nations have *uncontrolled* diabetes according to these standards (Casagrande, Fradkin, Saydah, Rust, & Cowie, 2013; Gakidou et al., 2011).

In prevention and treatment of diabetes, a key challenge is health behavior change. Medical interventions can partially alleviate or delay complications, but the course and outcomes of diabetes are heavily determined by patients' behavioral and lifestyle choices that are beyond the control of caregivers. Curricula for diabetes education focus on these health behavior changes that most patients find challenging to implement (Diabetes Control and Complications Trial Research Group, 1993; UKPDS Study Group, 1998). Yet, few health care professionals are trained in evidence-based methods for helping patients to change.

Much of health care, especially care for chronic conditions like diabetes, seems to operate from a deficit model aimed at providing people with what they are lacking. Diabetes medications appropriately compensate for metabolic deficits such as insulin insufficiency or resistance. Clearly needed behavior changes are often addressed in the same manner as a deficit in knowledge or motivation—the presumption being that patients don't change because they either don't know enough or care enough. This view

3

encourages providers to persuade patients to change by attempting to provide enough knowledge, insight, or fear to make a difference in how they
live their lives.

This book offers an alternative way of thinking about and addressing
the behavioral challenges of diabetes care. It is based on behavioral science
principles, and the specific method it describes—motivational interviewing
(MI)—now has a large evidence base of controlled clinical trials conducted
across many areas of health care. MI's application to diabetes care is more
recent, with most studies appearing since 2005. To be sure, there is still
much to learn in this area, but this book provides a starting point.

Ambivalence

Beyond its shock value, a new diagnosis of diabetes immediately presents
people with a daunting list of recommended lifestyle changes to make in the
long-term interest of their health:

- Eat more vegetables and cut carbohydrates.
- Decrease your fat intake to better manage lipid levels and weight.
- Regularly monitor your blood glucose levels.
- Increase your physical activity—exercise at least 150 minutes a
  week.
- Decrease your stress levels and avoid depression.
- Take your medications regularly, as prescribed.
- Monitor your blood pressure.
- Check your feet daily.
- Cut back on your drinking and stop smoking.
- Have regular eye exams.
- Visit your physician's office quarterly for medical check-ups.

The sheer volume of such changes and of new information can be overwhelming—even before considering the emotional impact of a diagnosis
that threatens one's life and well-being. This distress is further compounded
by the limited time that health care providers typically have with patients,
creating a great sense of urgency to meet all clinical practice guidelines
while also providing patients with solutions to these challenges.

Then there is the very human phenomenon of ambivalence. The status
quo is familiar and carries a certain inertia with it, whereas change requires
effort. One part of a patient wants to be healthy and knows that change is
needed, while another part may be comfortable with how things are and
therefore the patient is reluctant to make changes. Both arguments are con-
stantly at play within the patient.

Ambivalence is like having an internal control committee. There are members of the committee voicing the urgency and advantages of change, and there are conservative members who oppose it. Left to one's own devices, the patient usually listens to an argument from one side and then the other side for a bit, and then stops thinking about the matter altogether because such internal conflict is unpleasant. The stopping of debate means, of course, the status quo prevails, at least for the time being.

The Righting Reflex

Enter the helper, the health care worker who went into this profession with the desire to make a positive difference in the world and in the lives of others. When you see someone heading down a road that leads to suffering, you want to get right in front of that person and say: "Stop! Go back! Don't you see where this road leads? There is a much better way over there. Take that road instead." And you do this naturally and with the very best of intentions. It is, after all, part of your job to alleviate suffering. It's just a gut instinct, a reflex built into those of us who go into the helping professions. You naturally want to fix things. You want to make things right.

Now, consider what happens when someone who is ambivalent meets a time-pressured helper with the righting reflex. Remember that the ambivalent person has both prochange and counterchange voices on that internal committee. To illustrate, we will use the example of problem drinking, which is the area in which the method of MI originally began (Miller, 1983). The helper asks some questions about the patient's drinking, listens patiently, and after a few minutes says, "Well, I'm concerned that you have a serious drinking problem, and I recommend that you stop drinking, at least for a while."

You don't have to think hard to know what the patient's immediate response is likely to be: "No, I won't." There is nothing pathological or out of the ordinary about that. It's just human nature that whenever someone takes up one side of an ambivalent topic, a normal reaction is to voice the other side. Both views were already represented on the patient's internal committee, and the helper sided with one view. This could easily lead to a debate, with the helper defending the need for change and the patient defending the status quo. In a way, they would be acting out the patient's internal ambivalence.

That kind of interaction might be engaging, even therapeutic, except for another fact of behavioral science, namely, that people tend to believe their own arguments more than those of others. Experiments show that when people are caused (but not coerced) to argue on behalf of one perspective on an issue—even if it is opposite to their own prior position—their attitude and behavior tend to shift in that direction. People can literally talk themselves into (or out of) change.

Research bears out this last perception. When consultation sessions are recorded and coded, the likelihood of subsequent behavior change can be fairly accurately predicted by the levels of "change talk" (arguments for change) and "sustain talk" (arguments against change) that the patient voices spontaneously. The more change talk relative to sustain talk, the more likely change is to happen (Amrhein, Miller, Yahne, Palmer, & Fulcher, 2003; Moyers et al., 2007; Moyers, Martin, Houck, Christopher, & Tonigan, 2009). The more a patient argues against change, the less likely it is to occur.

So, there is the irony. When a helper tries to persuade an ambivalent patient by voicing the reasons for change, the patient's natural response is to argue against it (either overtly or silently while being passive). The more the patient voices the counterchange arguments, the less likely change becomes. Thus, persuasion can actually have the opposite effect of what was intended. It is the patient, not the helper, who should be voicing the arguments for change.

> *When a helper tries to persuade an ambivalent patient by voicing the reasons for change, the patient's natural response is to argue against it.*

Directing, Guiding, and Following

Now, we want to acknowledge that sometimes it *is* helpful for you to express your concern and offer advice from your professional expertise. When an antibiotic is needed, the physician gives clear instructions about how it should be taken ("Be sure to take this two times a day with food, and take all of the pills until they are gone—don't stop taking them as soon as you start to feel better."). Injured limbs can be fixed and warrant clear advice for self-care ("Keep the leg elevated, and don't put any weight on it for 10 days."). Giving information and advice reflects the clinical style of *directing*, and it is a natural part of health care, particularly in the treatment of acute conditions. Even when the goal is patient behavior change, directing sometimes works. A small proportion of smokers actually do quit smoking in response to simple physician advice, enough to make it worthwhile to try (Bao, Duan, & Fox, 2006; Lancaster & Stead, 2004).

At the opposite end of the spectrum is the clinical style of *following*—simply listening to your patient in an empathic, compassionate manner. By listening for a while, you may learn important things that you would not have discovered by reviewing a decision tree of questions. When you have done all you can to alleviate a dying patient's suffering, it is most humane just to listen for a while, following wherever the patient leads. Here it is the patient who provides the direction, and careful following on your part is another natural part of good health care.

In between these two extremes lies the interesting terrain of *guiding*. A good guide does not just bark orders. If you hire a guide in another country, he or she does not direct you as to when you will arrive and leave or what you will see. Rather, the guide's function is to understand what your interests are, what you would like to see and experience, and then to help you get there safely, efficiently, and enjoyably. To be sure, you rely on the guide for expertise, to offer direction as appropriate. You also rely on him or her to listen to you carefully (although a good guide doesn't merely follow you around). Guiding is a skillful blend of directing and following, resulting in expert guidance based on close listening.

> *Guiding is a skillful blend of directing and following.*

Neither directing nor following alone is very effective when what is needed is behavior change on the part of the patient. Often health care providers lean too heavily on directing, even for complex lifestyle and behavioral issues (Rollnick, Miller, & Butler, 2008). We find that the middle ground of guiding is most effective in helping patients to change their behavior.

Motivational Interviewing

MI is a refined form of guiding. It is a particular way of having a conversation about change, one that is designed to strengthen the patient's *own* motivations and commitment to change. MI is a way of helping patients voice their own reasons for change. When you find that you are arguing for change and your patient is arguing against it, you've got it exactly backwards from an MI perspective.

There is a definite direction to MI—it's not just following. You know where you hope to go, the change goal that you wish to reach. In that way, MI is different from the medical position of *equipoise*, in which you are consciously seeking *not* to influence the choice that a patient makes. MI is practiced to help patients move in a particular direction that is in their best interest. Usually it is the direction in which the patient has asked for help, and in which at least a *part* of the patient sees the need for change. MI is not a way of tricking patients into doing what you want or of persuading them to do what they are unwilling to do. Rather, it is a way of harnessing their own natural motivations for health and change.

Why Take Time to Learn This?

We sometimes receive invitations to teach MI in a 1- or 2-hour period. Unfortunately, that really can't be done! You can learn a bit *about* MI by attending a lecture or reading about it, but developing skillfulness in using the technique takes time and practice. It's less like learning a simple medical procedure and more like learning to play golf or a musical instrument in that you can keep getting better at it throughout your career.

So, why would you want to take the time and effort required to learn this complex skill? Because you are reading this book, we presume you are interested in helping your patients make changes that will benefit their health. With that assumption as a background, we suggest three reasons why you might choose to make the investment.

First of all, MI has a solid evidence base confirming its *efficacy*, with well over 200 randomized clinical trials published across a wide range of health behavior change issues (*www.guilford.com/add/miller2/biblio.pdf*). The largest evidence base thus far relates to alcohol/drug use (Hettema, Steele, & Miller, 2005; Jensen et al., 2011; Lundahl & Burke, 2009), but meta-analyses have also reported efficacy with smoking cessation (Lai, Cahill, Qin, & Tang, 2010), weight reduction (Armstrong et al., 2011), and in managing cholesterol and blood pressure (Rubak, Sandbaek, Lauritzen, & Christensen, 2005). Average effect sizes (relative to no intervention) have been in the small to medium range, with wide variability across studies, providers, and sites within multisite trials (Lundahl, Kunz, Brownell, Tollefson, & Burke, 2010).

In diabetes care, MI has been effective in lowering A1C levels in adolescents who have type 1 diabetes (T1D). Teenagers who received a series of individual counseling sessions using MI had significantly lower hemoglobin A1c levels than the control group, a difference still present a year after the study ended (Channon et al., 2007). MI has also been used successfully to help women with type 2 diabetes (T2D), though in this study African American women did not respond as well to MI as other women in the treatment group did (West, DiLillo, Bursac, Gore, & Greene, 2007).

MI appears to work across cultures well. Practitioners are being trained in at least 47 languages at present, and a meta-analysis found that MI had twice the effect size when delivered to U.S. minority populations (primarily Hispanic and African American) as compared to white-majority samples (Hettema et al., 2005).

A second reason to use MI is anecdotal, and one for which we hope to see solid research in the future—namely, the impact on clinicians themselves. Across health care, the corrections system, and addiction-related and mental health care, providers who learn MI often tell us that it makes their practice more *enjoyable*. A common theme is the lifting of a heavy burden—one related to the feeling of futility or personal responsibility to *make* patients change and to do it quickly. One of the quickest encouragements for their learning MI appears to be how readily patients respond even to their early approximations of MI.

Finally, MI is *learnable.* Here there is solid evidence from training studies, which have thus far found no relationship between years of education and the ability to learn MI (Miller, Yahne, Moyers, Martinez, & Pirritano, 2004). The skills are specifiable and can be reliably observed in practice. Once you know what to listen for, your patients can become your teachers because you receive immediate in-session feedback each and every time you practice MI. Some coaching and personal feedback can also improve skillfulness (Miller et al., 2004). Clinicians can learn how to influence the balance of change talk and sustain talk that their patients express, which in turn makes a difference in outcomes. The balance of patient change talk to sustain talk is clearly responsive to clinicians' MI skills (Glynn & Moyers, 2010; Moyers & Martin, 2006; Moyers, Miller, & Hendrickson, 2005; Vader, Walters, Prabhu, Houck, & Field, 2010).

Ultimately you decide how well this approach fits with your own practice style and in what ways it may benefit your patients. This book is designed to give you a clear introduction to and understanding of MI. Where you take it from there is up to you.

Key Points

- The effective management of diabetes requires a lot of behavior change for most patients.

- People tend to be ambivalent about change, with both pros and cons represented in their "internal committee."

- In an attempt to be helpful, health professionals often resort to the "righting reflex" and overly rely on a directing style.

- When someone advocates for change with a person who is ambivalent about it, a natural response is to defend the other side.

- MI is a learnable and evidence-based clinical style for helping patients to voice their own motivations for and ideas about change.

- MI is a refined form of guiding, which finds a middle road between directing and following.

CHAPTER 2

Mindset and Heartset

In the early years after MI was first introduced, training focused mostly on techniques. Clinicians came to workshops primarily for ideas about how to deal with "difficult" and "resistant" patients. As trainees began to apply MI techniques in their practice, however, it became apparent that something was very wrong. It was as if they had learned the words but not the music. The techniques seemed hollow, even manipulative, as if the clinician were trying to use tricks to outsmart the patient. Obviously, we were missing something important in our training.

What was missing, as it turned out, was the underlying spirit of MI (Rollnick & Miller, 1995), the state of mind and heart with which it is practiced. This is a set of basic presuppositions, a particular way of approaching people and the practice of MI. It is not essential to have internalized all of these assumptions before beginning to practice MI, however. If anything, the practice of a person-centered approach like MI seems to reinforce this way of being with people (Rogers, 1980). It is important, however, to understand this spirit as a context for practicing MI, and to be open to new habits of practice, much as the reader of a novel exercises what Samuel Taylor Coleridge called "the willing suspension of disbelief."

The Four Cornerstones

In the most recent description (Miller & Rollnick, 2013), the underlying mindset for the practice of MI rests on four foundational cornerstones. Here they are.

Partnership

You bring important expertise to your consultations, and so do your patients. They are the experts on themselves; no one knows more about them than they do. In short-term treatment of an acute condition, it may be less essential to draw on the patient's expertise, although even something as simple as taking an antibiotic requires that it be fit into the person's routine. When what

> *You bring important expertise to your consultations, and so do your patients. They are the experts on themselves.*

needs to change is the patient's lifestyle and behavior, however, that cannot be accomplished without collaboration. You bring your professional expertise, and patients bring what they know about themselves.

This fundamental perspective, then, is one of partnership. A conversation about change usually doesn't go well when one person acts like an expert for the other by advising, suggesting, and directing. Most people simply don't respond well to being told what to do, and as discussed in Chapter 1 there is a natural pushback that can even undermine change. The mindset here is that "we need to put our heads together" about how this could happen. It is not an expert talking down to a patient or a teacher to a student, but a person and a guide sorting out together how best to move ahead.

Acceptance

A second cornerstone is an attitude of acceptance of people as they are. This is not acquiescence or fatalism, but rather a mindful openness to what the person is experiencing. When people feel unacceptable, they find it difficult to change, dropping into a kind of behavioral paralysis. Ironically, it is when people experience being accepted as they are that it becomes possible for them to change (Rogers, 1959). To accept people as they are is to free them to change.

There are actually four components to this perspective, and they all begin with the letter *a*. First, people have *autonomy*: they get to make the choices about how they will live and what they will do. Much as one might be tempted to say, "You can't" or "You have to," the fact is that no one can take away this power of choice. It has to be OK with you that patients get to make the choices about their own behavior. This is not a matter of giving them something they did not already have. It is simply recognizing a reality, and this can be freeing for the clinician as well. You don't have to make choices about your patients' behavior or make them choose a particular path; you can't. Patients need to do that for themselves.

A second component of acceptance recognizes the *absolute worth* of every person. Patients don't have to prove their worth or earn your respect. They deserve dignity and humane treatment just by virtue of being human.

A third aspect is *accurate empathy*, the desire and effort to see the world from the patient's point of view. It is not sympathy or telepathy, but a practiced skill of understanding clearly what the patient is experiencing. This recognizes that there are perspectives other than your own, and that it is worth the effort to grasp what the patient perceives and means. We will say more about listening skills in Chapter 4.

Lastly, acceptance involves *affirmation* of the person's strengths and efforts. It is a conscious appreciation of what is good about this person. Every step taken in the right direction, no matter how small, is recognized and affirmed. Instead of catching and criticizing what people are doing wrong, you notice and appreciate what they are doing right. All of these aspects are part of an attitude of acceptance.

Compassion

The third cornerstone of the spirit of MI is *compassion*—the desire and intention to alleviate suffering, to seek the other's welfare, and of course to do no harm. This is perhaps the primary motivation that brings people into the helping professions. Compassion reminds us that the patient's well-being is our prime directive and the reason for our consultations. In the words of William Mayo, MD, in 1910, "The best interest of the patient is the only interest to be considered."

Evocation

The fourth and final cornerstone is *evocation*, a definitive component in the practice of MI. So much of medical practice has to do with inserting things into people. In MI the implicit message is not "I have what you need, and I'm going to give it to you," but rather "You have what you need, and together we will find it."

Now, again, you clearly have expertise to share. Diabetes education, for example, does involve conveying some important information. For patients to remember and use the information, however, it is vital that they be actively engaged in the education process. Monty Roberts (2001) observed that "there is no such thing as teaching; there is only learning" (p. xxii).

Using the perspective of ambivalence presented in Chapter 1, the MI practitioner assumes that at least a part of the person already *is* "motivated" for healthy change. There is a part of every smoker (sometimes just a small part) that knows smoking is self-destructive and wants to be free of it. In MI, you set out in search of that part—that ally within the patient. Your job is not to install motivation but to call forth that which is already there. We will say much more about this in the chapters to come.

Your job is not to install motivation but to call forth that which is already there.

A Firm Foundation

These four cornerstones provide a firm foundation for the practice of MI in diabetes care. They are the mindset and "heartset" behind patient care, the reason and context for using the clinical method presented in the rest of this book. MI is not fundamentally a technique or procedure. It is a way of being, a style of practice infused with the patient-centered perspective described above. To be sure, there is measurable technical proficiency involved; yet, it is as difficult to quantify the essence of MI as it is to specify what constitutes a skillful general practitioner.

We emphasize again that these attitudes are not prerequisites for learning how to practice MI. It remains to be seen how true you will experience them to be in your own work. Whatever your starting point, we hope you find material here that helps you to improve and enjoy your conversations with patients about change.

Key Points

- An important aspect of MI is the underlying mindset and heartset with which it is practiced.

- MI is a *partnership* in which helper and patient collaborate, each bringing his or her own expertise that is important in facilitating change.

- The MI practitioner manifests *acceptance* of people as they are, which ironically frees them to change.

- *Compassion* is a cornerstone of MI—a radical commitment to the patient's best interest.

- *Evocation*—to call forth the patient's own wisdom and ideas—differs from a deficit model of installing what the person is lacking (such as knowledge, insight, or motivation).

CHAPTER 3

Four Processes
of Motivational Interviewing

Over the years, much has evolved in how we understand and teach the clinical method of MI. One important step was gaining an appreciation for the underlying spirit with which MI is practiced (see Chapter 2). Foundational skills have been clarified (to be introduced in Chapter 4), and core principles defined (Miller & Rollnick, 1991, 2002). Today, we describe MI as having four core processes (Miller & Rollnick, 2013)—engaging, focusing, evoking, and planning—though all four do not necessarily occur within any particular consultation.

Engaging

Much has been written about the importance of developing rapport, a working relationship that facilitates communication and change. It is tempting for a clinician to charge right into the business at hand, particularly when time is short and other patients are waiting. This may suffice if you already have an established relationship of trust and communication with a particular patient. Too often, though, patients are left in the rather passive role of answering a few questions and waiting for a quick verdict. Diabetes education can too easily become a one-way information download. Lifestyle behavior change is unlikely to occur in this scenario precisely because change requires the clinician's active engagement of and collaboration with patients.

Providers try in different ways to develop rapport—a bit of small talk to start, asking a broad question, remembering a detail about the patient (perhaps from file notes checked before the consultation). Such niceties do help people relax but still do not actively engage them in their own care.

One key process in health care, particularly in chronic disease management, is patient activation (Hibbard, Mahoney, Stock, & Tusler, 2007), or having "a knowledgeable and activated patient as a collaborative partner in managing their health" (p. 1444). Rather than being a passive recipient of information and care, the patient is actively engaged in two-way communication and consultation with the clinician.

Engaging need not require a large amount of time at the outset. It can begin in minutes and is facilitated in part by the clinician's mindset (described in Chapter 2) communicated immediately to patients through particular practice behaviors that will be described in Chapter 4. Here is a brief example from a patient's follow-up visit with a diabetes educator.

CLINICIAN: Good morning, Jennifer. How are you, and how is your daughter?

PATIENT: She's fine, just starting school this year.

CLINICIAN: How exciting! They grow up so fast. I'm glad to see you coming back for follow-up visits like this. How are you doing in managing your diabetes? What's been going well, and what's been tough?

PATIENT: I'm taking my metformin most of the time; occasionally I forget it.

CLINICIAN: Good. That makes a real difference.

PATIENT: I see that, when I forget it, my glucose level goes way up.

CLINICIAN: That's interesting. Usually missing a single dose doesn't make much difference, but people do vary in how they respond. In any event you're checking your glucose levels, and that's important. How is that going for you?

PATIENT: There are times I don't want to test because of what I've eaten.

CLINICIAN: You already know it's going to be high, and don't want to see it.

It would be tempting to jump right in with advice, but the diabetes educator here is taking time to listen, to hear and understand the patient's perspective. A little engaging of this kind can provide a strong foundation for the other three MI processes.

In a primary care relationship, engagement can get a jump start at the beginning and then continue to grow over time. In one-time consultations it can be particularly important to devote conscious time for engagement at the outset before rushing into fact gathering or information sharing. In subsequent chapters, we offer further practical examples of how engaging can sound in clinical consultations.

Focusing

With adequate engagement, the next process is to develop a clear shared focus for the consultation, "What will we talk about today? What do we hope to accomplish?" In health care, this is usually established through the patient's presenting concerns. In diabetes care, a central goal is glycemic control, a disease management concern that patients may not adequately understand or share. To promote health and longevity, clinicians track key indicators with target ranges.

A variety of self-management behaviors contribute to glycemic control, so one aspect of focusing in diabetes care is *agenda setting*, choosing from a menu of options the behavioral topic or topics to discuss in this particular consultation. If you try to address all of the possible behavior changes at once, chances are that little or nothing will change.

A simple clinical tool used in MI is a bubble sheet, an example of which is shown in Figure 3.1. Though now widely used in other health care fields, this clinical tool was originally developed in diabetes care as a way for practitioners to help patients with uncontrolled T2D (Stott, Rees, Rollnick, Pill, & Hackett, 1996). In a typical consultation, after attending to any immediate concerns, the clinician might show the bubble sheet to the patient and say:

> "There are quite a few things people with diabetes can do to stay healthy, and I wonder which of these you might like to talk about today. For example, we could discuss physical activity or how you eat, checking your sugar level, managing stress, medications, or anything on this sheet—or perhaps there is something else you'd like to discuss. What do you think? Which one might be good for us to talk about today?"

Then there is the situation of a health topic that concerns you about this patient that you would like to discuss. Without offending the patient, how can you open up a potentially difficult topic that he or she has not raised? The key here is asking permission.

> "I notice that you are a smoker, and that is something with especially serious health consequences for people with diabetes. I'm not going to lecture you about it, but I wonder if you would be willing to talk about your smoking for a few minutes."

> "You know, I see that on the last few visits your A1c values have been increasing steadily, and I'm concerned. Would it be all right with you if we discuss this a bit?"

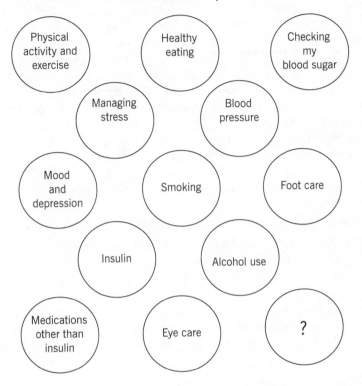

FIGURE 3.1. A sample bubble sheet.

Evoking

With an engaged patient and a clear focus, the next process is one that is fairly unique to and definitive of MI: evoking the person's *own* motivations for health and change. The righting reflex (as noted in Chapter 1) is to tell patients what they should do and why they should do it, particularly when you feel time-pressured. Physicians sometimes tell us, "I don't have *time* to do MI!" But if consultation time is brief and your goal is a patient's behavior change, then you can't afford *not* to try this approach because it is more likely to have the desired effect in a short time than is finger wagging, warning, or lecturing. MI is not an extended counseling process. A surprise in MI research has been how often and well it has worked in relatively brief contacts. (Meta-analyses of MI research are listed in the Appendix.)

> *It is the patient rather than the provider who should be voicing the arguments for change.*

As mentioned in Chapter 1, a core concept of MI is that *it is the patient rather than the provider who should be voicing the arguments for change.* The evoking process involves arranging your conversation so that this happens, and specific methods for doing so are discussed in Chapter 5. This also means restraining your well-intentioned righting reflex to provide the motivations and solutions yourself. Like diabetes management, MI requires some self-control in not doing the first thing that comes to mind. Here is a short example, even before we explain what the clinician is doing and why.

PATIENT: I'm just worried that my A1c value keeps going up. I don't like that.

CLINICIAN: And what is it that concerns you about that in particular?

PATIENT: I thought the medicine would help more, and I guess I don't want to have to go on insulin.

CLINICIAN: That worries you. Well, let me ask you this. How important would you say it is for you to get better control of your glucose levels, to get them down? Say, on a scale from 0 to 10, where 0 is not at all important, and 10 is the most important thing in your life right now, what number would you give yourself?

PATIENT: About a 6, I guess.

CLINICIAN: So, it's pretty important to you. Why a 6 and not, say, a 1 or 2?

PATIENT: You've told me the stuff that can happen with uncontrolled diabetes, and I don't want that.

CLINICIAN: What consequences are you remembering that would matter to you?

PATIENT: Well, I don't want to go blind. I love reading, and I couldn't do my work if I couldn't see.

CLINICIAN: Mm hmm. What else?

PATIENT: Kidney failure. Who wants to go on dialysis?

CLINICIAN: Those are things you definitely want to avoid.

In this example, it is the patient who is making the arguments for change, and that is no accident. Neither is it because this is a particularly "motivated" patient. Such natural evoking happens by the way in which the clinician conducts the conversation.

Planning

The evoking process helps to strengthen patients' own motivation to make a change. When the person seems sufficiently willing to consider change, then (and only then) is it time for the fourth process: planning. If you jump into the how and when of change too soon, before enough consideration has been given to whether and why, you are likely to run into reluctance and inaction.

> *If you jump into the how and when of change too soon, you are likely to run into reluctance and inaction.*

Now, some patients do occasionally come into your office ready for change. A new diagnosis of diabetes may have lighted a fire under them to take charge and get healthy. For such patients there's no great need for evoking, spending a lot of time pondering whether and why. They are already past that point and want to talk about how to make necessary changes for their health. For them, planning is the main task. Of course, it also happens that, once you get into planning, ambivalence can rear its head and you need to double back to engaging, focusing, and evoking.

Planning, by the way, is not just a one-time event. It is a process of working out long-term self-care strategies, and plans usually need adjusting along the way. Each plan is provisional—something to try out to see how it works. Planning is also not the time for you to grab the reins and provide the answers, much as you might want to do that. Like all of MI, planning is a collaborative process combining your expertise and the patient's.

The goal in such collaboration is to come up with a self-care plan that the patient accepts and will implement. This is where you particularly need patients' self-knowledge about what is realistic, what will be possible and workable in their daily lives. The plan should not be vague and general ("I will get my blood sugar under better control") but specific enough to implement. Often the plan is simply the most logical next step on the road to glycemic control. Here are some examples of specific plans that a patient might decide to try:

> "I will start out checking my blood sugar first thing in the morning and 2 hours after meals, and keep a record."
>
> "I plan to keep track of what I eat and try to have no more than four carbs [of 15 grams] in each meal."
>
> "If I snack in between meals, I am going to stick to a serving of nuts or a piece of fruit."
>
> "I intend to exercise for 50 minutes on Monday, Wednesday, and Friday evenings."

Don't worry too much about everything that could go wrong with the plan. It will surely need some adjusting over time. The point is to get to a starting plan to which the patient can say "Yes" and then (as your setting allows) check back over time. (Follow-up visits in diabetes care are discussed in Chapter 11.)

What is involved in a patient saying "Yes"? Research on implementation intentions (Gollwitzer, 1999) shows that people are much more likely to follow through when they state a *specific* plan and their *intention* to carry it out. All of the above examples of specific plans are also implementation intentions when stated to another person because they contain language that signals a commitment: "I will," "I intend to," "I am going to," "I plan to." Don't pressure patients to say such words if they don't seem ready. Ideally, a planning process leads naturally to the spontaneous expression of such intention. If you wonder, you can always ask when you hear a specific plan:

"So is that what you're going to do?"
"Sounds like a good plan. Are you willing to do that, then?"

although we do not recommend exerting undue pressure for commitment:

"So, are you going to do it or not?"

Must I Do the Processes in Order?

In theory, the four processes are somewhat linear. It is hard to make much progress on change if you fail to engage with your patient, so that is a first step. Before you can evoke, you must know what your focus is—the direction of change toward which you hope to move—because change talk can only be recognized in relation to a particular change goal. Typically, it is not time for specific planning until a sufficient motivational foundation has been laid. "Whether" and "why" questions tend to come before "how" and "when."

In practice, however, we don't experience such unidirectional straight-line movement in MI. Sometimes the focus is predetermined by the practice setting (e.g., a smoking cessation clinic) or the patient's priorities even before engagement occurs. Evoking and change talk may occur in the first few minutes of a consultation. The focus of consultation can change over time. An attempt to start planning may reveal a need to double back and do more evoking, clarifying of focus, or even engaging.

Thus, MI is definitely not about marching through the four processes in order. Attending and responding to the patient's experience in the present moment is much more important than adhering to any formula or guideline for the practice of MI. Listening to your patient tells you where you are within the processes and where to go next.

Following this overview of the spirit (Chapter 2) and processes of MI, we now proceed to practical skills. We begin in Chapter 4 with the four foundational communication microskills for engaging, the same skills that are used throughout the practice of MI. Then, in Chapter 5, we apply these microskills in particular ways for evoking patient motivation for change.

Key Points

- MI can be understood as four integrated processes.

- *Engaging* requires understanding the patient's point of view as a way to develop a working alliance with him or her.

- *Focusing* is the process of developing one or more clear goals for change.

- *Evoking* calls forth the patient's own motivations for and ideas about change.

- *Planning* involves the collaborative development of the next steps that the patient is willing to take.

CHAPTER 4

OARS

Four Foundational Practice Skills

The skills presented in this chapter provide a foundation for clear communication, not only in professional consultation but in relationships more generally. They derive from the well-established tradition of person-centered counseling and medicine (Egan, 2013; Gordon & Edwards, 1997; Rogers, 1965). These skills facilitate rapid engagement, giving the patient an immediate active role in the consultation. The same skills are used throughout the MI processes and are applied in specific ways in the process of evoking (discussed in Chapter 5).

The four microskills are represented by the mnemonic acronym OARS: open questions, affirming, reflecting, and summarizing. The OARS are tools for creating momentum through the waters of change.

Asking Open Questions

Health care professionals are accustomed to asking questions to collect patient information and then proceed down decision trees to reach a diagnosis. Most of their questions need only a short answer, such as:

Yes or no	"Are you allergic to any medications?"
A number	"What is your pain level, on a scale from 0 to 10?"
A fact	"What is your address?"
A date or time	"When did you first notice the blurry vision?"
A name	"What is the blood pressure medicine that you are taking?"

Short-answer questions like these are called *closed* questions. They restrict the range of likely answers and thus can be efficient for collecting specific information in a short time. Asking a series of short-answer questions quickly places the patient in a passive role—"I ask the questions, and you give the answers"—and it puts the clinician in a one-up power position. That is not always bad—it's just what happens when someone is asked a series of rapid-fire questions. It also implies that when you are done asking the questions, you will have an answer. That may be the case with a diagnosis or prescription, but when it comes to lifestyle behavior changes the answers must involve the patient.

Open questions, in contrast, give the person being questioned more room to respond. They do not invite a short answer, and it is harder to guess what the reply will be.

> "What brings you in today?"
>
> "Tell me how you've been feeling since I saw you last."
>
> "What has been the biggest challenge for you in managing your diabetes?"
>
> "How is your family doing?"
>
> "How do you think you could best remember to check your blood levels?"

Such questions prompt patients to search their memory banks and tell you what is on their mind. With open questions, you can also get information that you might otherwise miss with closed questions. Open questions put the patient in a more active participatory role. They feel less like an interrogation and more like a conversation.

> *Open questions put the patient in a more active participatory role.*

Sometimes busy practitioners are nervous about open questions, feeling less in control and worrying about opening up a Pandora's box by allowing too much latitude for the patient to talk. Nevertheless, open questions are more likely to invite patient engagement, honesty, comfort, and active participation. Straying too far off-track can usually be prevented with a gentle redirection:

> "So, let me come back to what we were talking about before."
>
> "I understand. Now here's what I would like to do next."

Here are some examples of open questions that you might ask in a first consultation with a person who has diabetes:

"How did you first discover that you have diabetes?"

"In what ways has your diabetes been a problem or limitation for you?"

"What have you been doing so far to manage your blood sugar?"

"Tell me what you already know about the HbA1c blood test."

"How do you hope I might be able to help you with your health?"

Such questions open the door for a conversation about health and self-care. Open questions offer a way of getting the conversation started.

Affirming

A second important tool in facilitating communication is *affirming*. An affirmation comments positively on a patient's qualities, strengths, and efforts. It is a statement of appreciation, and it should be both truthful and sincere. People often fear bad news when coming for health care, having to face learning what is *wrong* with them. To affirm is to celebrate what is *right* with them.

Affirmation builds relationship. It's rare enough to hear positive comments! Affirming also tends to put people at ease and to decrease defensiveness. There is less need to defend when you are being appreciated rather than attacked. Affirming fosters engagement.

Although it's easy to get out of the habit of affirming, it's simple enough to do. One form is appreciation of positive action:

"Thanks for bringing in these records of your sugar levels. That's very helpful."

"I'm glad you came in to have this looked at."

"I see you had your blood test drawn. Good!"

"I like how you said that!"

"Running three times a week. That's terrific!"

You can also chain together affirmations and open questions:

"Your A1c level is down, so you must be doing something right. What have you changed?"

"I'm glad you're exercising more. How is that going for you?"

Other affirmations focus on a personal characteristic or strength:

"You've been sticking with this. When you put your mind to something, you get it done!"

"Your children are really important to you."
"You've been patient through a lot of changes—I appreciate that."
"You really care about your health!"

Reflecting

Reflecting, also called "active listening," is a particular way of responding to what patients tell you. It helps ensure that you understand what patients mean, and also serves as a mirror for patients to reflect on their own situation. Reflection is an important skill in MI, and it's one that takes a while to develop. Those who are good at reflecting make it look easy, but it's actually harder than it appears at first.

Here is how it works. Before a person says anything, there is something that he or she is experiencing in that moment, what he or she *means* to communicate. The person puts this into words, and that's the first place where communication can go wrong since people don't always say what they mean. You could mishear the words, but even if you hear them correctly you still have to make a guess about what the person means. Thus, your interpretation of meaning actually could be three steps removed from what the person actually meant. Most people most of the time respond to their interpretation as if it *were* what the person meant, and so communication can go awry quickly.

A reflective listening statement, the key skill to learn here, makes a *guess* about the speaker's meaning. Rather than assuming you already know, it is a way of checking to see if you have it right by offering a short summary of what you heard, often in somewhat different words.

PATIENT: I just hate sticking my finger to check my sugar.

CLINICIAN: It really hurts. (Reflection)

PATIENT: Well, not all that much. It's more the expectation.

CLINICIAN: Holding the lancing device and waiting to push it. (Reflection)

PATIENT: Yes! I think that's worse than the stick itself.

Notice what is *not* happening here. First of all, the clinician is not jumping straight into a righting reflex problem-solving role:

PATIENT: I just hate sticking my finger to check my sugar.

CLINICIAN: Let me show you how to do it so it won't hurt as much.

Second, the practitioner is not just repeating what the patient said, which gets boring in a hurry:

PATIENT: I just hate sticking my finger to check my sugar.

CLINICIAN: You hate sticking your finger.

Instead, it is like they are constructing a paragraph together. Third, the clinician is not asking questions:

PATIENT: I just hate sticking my finger to check my sugar.

CLINICIAN: Does it hurt a lot?

What the clinician *is* doing is taking a moment to understand what the patient means, to get inside his or her experience of self-care. It doesn't have to take much time. In fact, it sometimes takes less time, and patients know that you "get" them—that you understand their perspective.

So how do you do this? There are just two guidelines:

1. Make your response a statement, not a question. Remove any question words (e.g., "Are you . . . ?" "Do you mean . . . ?" "Is it . . . ?), and also inflect your voice *downward* at the end of the statement ("It really hurts."). If you inflect upward ("It really hurts?"), it's still a question.
2. Make a guess about what the person means. The fact that you are guessing may make you want to ask it as a question instead, but it's better to offer your response as a statement, as questions tend to put people on the defensive.

It takes a while to get the hang of this, but it's worth putting in the effort. Skillful reflection is a very quick way to establish rapport. It helps patients to process their own experience and to know that you understand them. It decreases miscommunication and strengthens clinician–patient relationship. Besides all that, you are

> *Skillful reflection is a very quick way to establish rapport.*

likely to learn things you would otherwise have missed. You also get immediate feedback every time you offer a reflection, and it doesn't matter if your guess was right or wrong. Either way people tell you more about what they meant.

Here is another example from a diabetes consultation. Most of the clinician's responses are reflections.

CLINICIAN: Tell me what you've been doing to get your glucose levels down. (Open question)

PATIENT: I've been trying to watch what I eat, and that's hard.

CLINICIAN: It's a challenge for you. (Reflection)

PATIENT: Yes. I know I should avoid carbohydrates, but I just crave them.

CLINICIAN: You've got a sweet tooth. (Reflection—making a guess)

PATIENT: No, it's not sweets so much as things that go crunch: crackers, potato chips, pretzels, breakfast cereal. And I love bread.

CLINICIAN: And you understand the problem with those foods for you. (Reflection)

PATIENT: My body turns them right into sugar.

CLINICIAN: Right, exactly! (Affirmation) So, what strategies have you found so far that seem to work for you? (Open question)

PATIENT: Well, not buying those things—not having them around the house.

CLINICIAN: That's a good strategy! (Affirmation) What else? (Open question)

PATIENT: I cut up carrots and fresh fruit and keep it in the fridge for snacks.

CLINICIAN: For those times when you feel a twinge of hunger. (Reflection)

PATIENT: Yes. If it's already prepared, then I'll take that, especially if I don't have junk food around.

CLINICIAN: That's a one-two combination that seems to work for you: avoid having junk food around, and make it easy to eat healthier snacks. (Summary reflection)

In one minute of conversation the clinician has a clearer sense of what this patient is doing so far. The conversation could stop here or continue with "What else?" As will become clearer in Chapter 5, it also matters that it is the *patient* who is voicing self-care strategies. Once the clinician understands what the person is already doing, he or she might then transition into offering a suggestion (discussed further in Chapter 6).

Summarizing

The fourth microskill within OARS is offering summaries. These draw together things that the *patient* has said. Of course, it's also possible to give a reminder summary of what you have said, but here it is the patient's own content that is being summarized. In this way, a summary is like a reflection, offering back your understanding of what the person has been saying.

It collects material from earlier in the conversation, or even from a prior consultation, and pulls it all together.

Summaries can be short, offered along the way. The above dialogue ended with an example of this, pulling together the two strategies that the patient had voiced so far. Summaries can also be a bit longer, collecting what has been said in a conversation as you transition to another task. For example:

> "The things that concern you most, then, about having uncontrolled diabetes are longer-term disabilities like blindness, amputation, or needing dialysis. You definitely would like to avoid those complications. Right now you feel pretty healthy, and you'd like to stay that way. [Summary] So let's talk about what might be some next steps to stay healthy. [Transitioning to planning]"

Summarizing is affirming because it shows that you are listening and remembering what the patient says. It communicates, "I hear you, and what you say is so important that I remember it and put the pieces together." Summaries also help patients to integrate what they are experiencing in health care and self-care. They voice their experience, then they hear you reflect it, and later they hear it again in a summary. It sounds like this might take a long time, but it can occupy only a few minutes, and it is sometimes surprising how much ground is covered in that time as you become skilled in reflecting and summarizing.

The OARS skills fit together nicely, as illustrated in the dialogues above and in subsequent chapters. The skillful practitioner weaves them together in a natural conversational style, but it's not just chat. As we will see in the next chapter, specific things are happening within such conversations.

Key Points

- Four communication skills (represented by the mnemonic acronym OARS) are used throughout the processes of MI.

- *Open questions* give the patient latitude in how to respond.

- *Affirmations* emphasize the patient's strengths, positive attributes, and efforts.

- *Reflections* offer a short summary of something a patient has said, making a guess about its meaning.

- *Summaries* pull together important pieces of what a patient has said.

CHAPTER 5

Hearing, Evoking, and Responding to Change Talk

The language of change is fascinating, and you are already at least somewhat familiar with it just by virtue of living in society and relating to others. For example, when you ask someone to do something for you, you listen carefully to what the person says in response because it contains clues about whether he or she will actually do it. Consider the different shades of meaning in these possible replies to your request:

"I would be glad to do it for you."
"I think I can do that."
"I wish I could."
"I'll try to get to it."
"I'll take care of it right away."
"I owe it to you."
"I'd like to, but I'm not sure I can."

Sensitivity to language is a key in any negotiation process, and that includes the particular kind of conversation about change that MI represents.

When considering a new action, people can in essence talk themselves into or out of doing it (Miller & Rollnick, 2004). Successful salespeople know this very well (Cialdini, 2007). The "talking" isn't necessarily spoken aloud. Sometimes it is private self-talk in thought or written form, but often conversation with others has a substantial impact on decisions.

In thinking about a possible change, most people have both pros and cons; they can voice arguments both for and against making the change. That is the nature of ambivalence: part of the person (some portion of their "internal committee") favors the change, and another part opposes it or at least is more reluctant. An ambivalent person can verbalize arguments for either side, or both. As discussed in Chapter 1, if someone else takes up one side of this internal argument, the ambivalent person is likely to respond by advocating for the opposite side.

In MI, people's own motivations for making a change are termed, simply enough, *change talk*, whereas their motivations to maintain the status quo and not change are called *sustain talk*. Almost all MI research has focused on change talk and sustain talk as spoken aloud by patients during consultation, but these forms of speech can also happen as covert self-talk or in writing (Miller, 2014). From this research it is clear that it *matters* what patients say. Change is less likely to happen when patients express more sustain talk than change talk. In contrast, when the pros outweigh the cons in patients' speech, change is more likely to occur (Barnett et al., 2014; Bertholet, Faouzi, Gmel, Gaume, & Daeppen, 2010; Miller & Rollnick, 2004; Moyers et al., 2009).

> *Change is less likely to happen when patients express more sustain talk than change talk.*

"Well, of course!" you say. "Those patients who are more motivated are the ones who are going to change." And that's precisely where you would be stuck—as a helpless passive observer of patients' motivation levels—except for another important fact borne out in many studies, that providers can and do substantially influence the balance of change talk and sustain talk that patients express (Glynn & Moyers, 2010; Moyers & Martin, 2006). The easiest way to verify this is to voice to your patients the reasons why you think they should change and how they could do it. The result is likely to be patients' sustain talk: reluctance, backpedaling, or passivity, followed by little or no change.

So is MI, then, just a slick kind of reverse psychology—where you argue against change, causing the patient to argue for it? Not at all. Most people quickly see through that kind of manipulation and resent it. Rather, MI is about helping people to express and explore their own change talk, their own motivations to make a change that is in their self-interest—in this case, to manage better their own glucose levels to promote greater length and quality of life. Arranging your consultation conversations in this way to help people find their own motivations for change is a conscious and quite skillful process.

Recognizing Change Talk

A first step, then, is to "tune" your ear to hear change talk, to notice it when it occurs and recognize it as significant. Of all the things that patients say to you, change talk should stand out as particularly important, a signal that guides what you should say and do next. Change talk *matters*.

Psycholinguistic studies have helped us to distinguish between two kinds of change talk: *preparatory* and *mobilizing*. *Preparatory* change talk signals that the person is thinking about change, "getting ready" to consider it, but not yet decided. As the name implies, *mobilizing* change talk, on the other hand, signals movement toward change. The person is getting closer. These are not peculiar forms of speech but rather ones that people express and encounter almost every day.

Preparatory Change Talk

Four common but different types of speech acts illustrate preparatory change talk, although this is by no means an exhaustive list. If a patient says something that feels to you like it favors change, it probably is change talk whether or not it fits into any of our example categories. Intuitively recognizing change talk is a normal and important skill for living in community with others.

Desire

The first example of preparatory change talk is speech that indicates a desire signaled by using words such as *want*, *wish*, and *like*. Every language on the face of the earth has a way of expressing this.

> "I want to lose some weight."
> "I wish I could get my A1c level down."
> "I would like to exercise more."
> "I would prefer not to have to go on insulin."
> "I hate sticking my finger."

Notice in this last example that the very same form of speech can be sustain talk favoring the status quo:

> "I don't want to go on a strict diet."
> "I just love chocolate!"
> "I enjoy being able to eat whatever I like."
> "I hate exercising."

It is normal to hear both of these types of statements from ambivalent people: "I want to, and I don't want to." That's what ambivalence is. Both are true simultaneously, and there is nothing abnormal about that. Ambivalence is human nature.

Ability

A second kind of preparatory change talk relates to the person's perceived capability of changing, signaled in words such as *could*, *can*, and *able*.

"I think I *could* quit smoking."
"I might be *able* to lose 20 pounds."
"It would be *possible* for me to fit in more exercise."
"I *can* remember to take my medication on time."
"I *know how* to keep my blood sugar level down."

Ability is different from desire. The person speaking any of the above sentences might not *want* to change, and certainly is not saying that he or she will—just that it's possible. On the other side of the scale, ability is also a theme in sustain talk:

"I just *can't* quit smoking. I've failed several times."
"I *can* eat whatever I want."
"I don't know how I *could* possibly fit in any more time for exercise."

Reasons

A third form of preparatory change talk specifies a reason. It has an "if–then" structure, at least implicitly: if I do this, then that would happen.

"I'm sure I'd have more energy if I lost some weight."
"I certainly don't want to go blind [by not controlling my diabetes]."
"Exercising would also help me look more attractive."

And again, a stated reason can favor the status quo:

"I live alone, and I'm afraid if I go on insulin my sugar will go low and I won't wake up."
"I'm already not spending enough time with my kids, even without exercising."
"Checking my sugar levels all the time just makes me nervous."

Need

Our final example of preparatory change talk is a statement of need. A need statement has an imperative quality or urgency to it, without necessarily specifying why. It might contain words like *have to*, *need to*, *got to*, or *must*.

"I *have to* do something about my A1c level."
"I've *got to* start eating better."
"I *need to* exercise more."

And sustain talk also takes this form on behalf of the status quo:

"I don't *need to* quit smoking."
"I don't *have to* check my sugar level all the time."
"I *must* get off of these medications."

We use the mnemonic acronym DARN to remember these four types of preparatory change talk: Desire, Ability, Reasons, and Need. Notice that preparatory change talk does not say or imply that "I will"—that is the main way in which it differs from mobilizing change talk.

"I want to" does not mean that it's going to happen.
"I could" does not imply "I will."
A reason is often not enough to motivate change.
And even "I have to" is not the same as "I am going to."

Mobilizing Change Talk

Mobilizing change talk signals movement—that the person's ambivalence is beginning to resolve in the direction of change. We have identified three types as examples of mobilizing change talk with the acronym CATs: Commitment, Activation, and Taking steps.

Commitment

Committing language implies an agreement, and a strong form is also the simplest, "I will." This is the response you hope to hear when you ask a person to do something. It is also the language of contracts. There are stronger forms:

"Yes, I am going to."
"I will."
"I promise."
"I guarantee."

and somewhat weaker forms:

"I intend to."
"I hope to."
"I probably will."

Activation

This form of change talk is not quite a commitment, but it does signal movement. Some sample language is *ready to, prepared to,* and *willing to.*

"I am *willing* to start monitoring my blood sugar."
"I am *ready* to increase my exercise."

"I am *prepared* to start on insulin."
"I will *think about* quitting smoking."

Such language would not be sufficient commitment for most legal contracts, at the marriage altar, or in response to a swearing-in question in court: "Do you solemnly swear to tell the truth, the whole truth, and nothing but the truth?" Nevertheless, activation language signals that the person is getting closer to committing.

Taking Steps

A third type of mobilizing change talk became apparent in listening to MI consultations. It describes something that the person has already done—a step in the direction of change:

"I filled the prescription you gave me."
"I started checking my sugar every morning."
"I bought a pair of running shoes."
"I got rid of all the junk food in my house."

Such actions do not constitute a commitment, but they do predict longer-term change.

As with preparatory language, mobilizing language can also be uttered in the service of the status quo:

"I am going to keep on smoking." (Commitment)
"I am not willing to give up chocolate." (Activation)
"I tore up the prescription you gave me." (Taking steps)

So, tune up your ear to listen for change talk and sustain talk, because they matter. Furthermore, whenever you hear change talk, it is a signal that you're on the right track. If you hear a lot of sustain talk, it is the patient telling you to try something different from what you were just doing.

Evoking Change Talk

You don't have to wait in hopes that your patient will express some change talk. It does happen spontaneously, but there are also strategies you can use to evoke it, increasing the amount and strength of change talk that you will hear.

Perhaps the simplest and most common strategy for increasing patient change talk is to *ask for it*. Ask an open question the answer to which is likely to be change talk.

> "Why would it be important for you to get your diabetes under control?"
> "What do you already know about the consequences of uncontrolled diabetes?"

To elicit preparatory change talk, we use the acronym DARN to generate possible questions:

> "What do you hope for your own health in the future?" (Desire)
> "What one step might you be able to take to control your blood sugar better?" (Ability)
> "What would you say are three good reasons to manage your diabetes well?" (Reasons)
> "What do you think you need to do at this point?" (Need)

Another good way of inquiring about Need is to ask about the importance of change. For this, we use a 0–10 rating scale: "On a scale from 0 to 10, where 0 is 'not at all important' and 10 is 'the most important thing in my life right now,' how important would you say it is for you to get your diabetes well controlled?" It is a closed question the answer to which is a number, and that number is the starting point for this follow-up question: "And why are you at a _____ and not 0?" Notice that the answer to that question would normally be change talk. *Don't* ask why the person is at their number and not a higher one! The answer to that is sustain talk, all the reasons why it's not so important.

It is also possible to ask CATs questions, though be careful not to be too pushy in doing so (e.g., "Well, are you going to do it or not?"). Usually patients explore preparatory change talk before they come around to mobilizing change talk.

> "What have you already done to get better control of your diabetes?" (Taking steps)
> "What might you be willing to do as a next step?" (Activation)
> "So, what do you think you'll do?" (Commitment)

Beyond directly asking evoking questions there are other ways to get change talk started (Miller & Rollnick, 2013). One of them is looking ahead and anticipating the consequences of status quo and change. This is not you telling patients what to expect, but rather asking them what they anticipate. Remember that the intention is to evoke change talk, and if you make the arguments for change yourself, you're likely to get the opposite. Here are some examples of looking ahead:

> "If you don't make any more changes in managing your diabetes, what do you think your life might be like 5 years from now?"
> "How would you like for your health to be 5 or 10 years down the line? . . . And what do you think you can do to help that happen?"

A related option is to explore what the person cares most about. In a cardiac rehabilitation program with patients who had had a heart attack (Scales, Lueker, Atterbom, Handmaker, & Jackson, 1997), the primary motivator was usually not fear of death but rather reasons for living. There are many ways to open up this topic:

> "What do you look forward to most in the next 10 years?"
> "What are you enjoying most about being alive?"
> "What are the best reasons for you to stay healthy and well in the years ahead?"

In sum, find ways to arrange your consultation conversations so that your patients tell you why and how they might want, be able to, or have reason to or need to manage their diabetes better. You can also offer your own expertise (which we discuss in the next chapter), but nothing motivates like talking oneself into change. As the French philosopher Blaise Pascal observed, "People are generally better persuaded by the reasons which they have themselves discovered than by those which have come into the mind of others."

Responding to Change Talk

Getting change talk started is just the beginning. When you hear change talk, don't just let it pass by ("OK, what else?"). Become interested and curious to hear more about it.

As we listen to consultations, we hope that when we hear change talk the clinician will follow up with one of four specific responses. You already encountered them in Chapter 4: OARS—open questions, affirmations, reflection, and summaries. Here we put them to work to move in the direction of change.

First, when you hear change talk, you can ask more about it. Use an *open question* to ask for elaboration or an example:

PATIENT: I just want to be healthier.

CLINICIAN: *In what ways* would you like to be healthier?

PATIENT: I feel like my diabetes is really limiting me, like a handicap.

CLINICIAN: *Give me an example* of how this disease is interfering with your life.

PATIENT: I could probably do more to keep my sugar levels down.

CLINICIAN: What comes to mind? What might be three things you could do?

Second, *affirm* change talk when you hear it.

PATIENT: Maybe I could cut out having cold cereal for breakfast. That seems to drive up my sugar.

CLINICIAN: That sounds like a good idea!

PATIENT: I bought a pair of running shoes this week.

CLINICIAN: Good for you!

PATIENT: I want to be around to see my grandchildren grow up.

CLINICIAN: Your family is very important to you.

This last clinician response can also be considered a *reflection*, which is a third way to respond when you hear change talk.

PATIENT: It's hard for me to change how I eat, but I know that I need to.

CLINICIAN: You know how much of a difference it makes in your health.

PATIENT: I might be able to fit in some exercise after the kids have gone to bed.

CLINICIAN: That seems challenging but possible for you.

PATIENT: When my sugar goes so high, it scares me.

CLINICIAN: It really worries you to see that much of a spike.

Finally, you can respond to change talk with a *summary*. A particularly good way to do this is to summarize all the change talk themes that you have heard, putting them together like a bouquet of flowers that you offer to the patient.

PATIENT: And I just don't want to keep seeing my A1c level creeping up each time I come in. That's really discouraging.

CLINICIAN: (*summarizing what the patient has previously said*) So what you're thinking about doing is making some significant changes in how you eat, particularly cutting down carbohydrates like the breakfast cereal that seems to drive your blood sugar up.

You really don't like it when it jumps up like that. You've been doing well with monitoring, and you plan to keep that up. And the other thing is stepping your exercise up a notch, and you think you could try fitting that in after the kids go to bed.

That's a complete package. You ask open questions to get change talk going. Then, as it emerges, you respond with OARS. Patients hear themselves saying it; you reflect so they hear their own motivations again; you are interested and ask more; then you pull it all together in a summary, and they hear their own words once more. It can have quite a powerful impact.

We conclude this chapter with a dialogue illustrating how these strategies can be brought together in a consultation. Before doing so, however, there is one more topic to address.

Responding to Sustain Talk

When working with people who are ambivalent, you will naturally hear both change talk and sustain talk. We have explained how to evoke and respond to change talk, but what about sustain talk? Should you just ignore it? No. There can be important information in patients' sustain talk, and if you ignore it they may just repeat it because you don't seem to have heard it. You don't have to go excavating for sustain talk, but when patients do express it (and of course they will), here are some guidelines for responding.

First of all, resist the righting reflex to disagree, refute, or persuade. That is most likely to result in more sustain talk:

PATIENT: I hate sticking my finger for blood. It hurts for hours afterward.

CLINICIAN: It's just a little stick, and it shouldn't really hurt that much.

PATIENT: But it does. My ring finger here is still sore from this morning.

CLINICIAN: You could use a new lancet each time. You know how to change it?

PATIENT: Yes, but it doesn't help that much, and it gets kind of expensive.

CLINICIAN: Well, I can show you how to adjust the scale on the lancing device. You might not have it set right, and it hurts because it is going in too deep.

PATIENT: No, I've tried that. I already know how to adjust it. I just have sensitive fingers.

"Yes, but . . . " is the normal response when you disagree or try to correct sustain talk. It may feel like the natural thing to do (righting reflex), but the most common result when you push back is more sustain talk.

So, what *are* some better ways to respond? A good default is to *reflect* sustain talk. It shows that you are listening, heard what the person said, and are not disapproving or criticizing.

PATIENT: My feet are just fine. I don't need to be checking them every day.

CLINICIAN: You're not really worried about your feet.

PATIENT: Sometimes I just stop monitoring for weeks at a time.

CLINICIAN: As if it's better not to know. (Continuing the paragraph)

PATIENT: I can't believe how much I have to do to keep on top of this.

CLINICIAN: It just seems overwhelming sometimes, and yet you do it!

PATIENT: No, I don't want to think about starting on insulin.

CLINICIAN: That seems like too big a step for you.

PATIENT: When I eat the wrong things I just take more insulin.

CLINICIAN: That's how you plan to stay healthy.

It is important that such reflections are offered with no hint of sarcasm. As you might imagine, the very same words can have quite a different impact, depending on your tone of voice. If you voice these reflections in a way that communicates disagreement or cynicism, you're likely to engender more sustain talk and defensiveness on the part of the patient. Here's a place where the underlying spirit of MI is important: partnership, acceptance, compassion, and evocation comes into play. Remember that you *do* get to voice any concerns you may have (as you will see in the next chapter). When you're reflecting sustain talk, however, the purpose is to make sure that you fully understand what the patient means and to communicate that understanding back to the patient.

Oddly enough, we find that when we reflect sustain talk, the patient's next response can often be change talk.

PATIENT: My feet are just fine. I don't need to be checking them every day.

CLINICIAN: You're not really worried about your feet.

PATIENT: Well, sure, I don't want to have problems with my feet. (Change talk) I just never have seen anything of concern when I do check.

CLINICIAN: Good for you! So, you do check your feet sometimes; it's just that every day seems unnecessary.

PATIENT: That's right.

CLINICIAN: So, how often do you think it might be reasonable for you to check your feet—because, like, you and I don't want any surprises there.

PATIENT: Maybe once a week? Is that enough?

CLINICIAN: I'd feel better if you checked a bit more often, but of course it's up to you.

This last clinician response is an example of another theme in responding to sustain talk: supporting patients' autonomy and emphasizing their personal choice and control. This can vex one's righting reflex, but it is the truth. It really *is* the patient who gets to make the decisions about what to do. Emphasizing that freedom has a way of taking the wind out of the sails of reluctance. If you emphasize people's freedom of choice, then they don't have to.

PATIENT: I just don't like exercising. In fact, I hate it.	*Sustain talk*
CLINICIAN: And it is your choice whether and how you will be physically active. Nobody can make that choice for you. So, on a scale from 0 to 10, where 0 is not at all important and 10 is extremely important, how important would you say it is for you to increase your physical activity in order to manage your diabetes and prevent complications?	*Emphasizing personal choice* *Open evocative question, using the importance ruler*
PATIENT: I don't know. Five, maybe.	
CLINICIAN: Five. So, somewhat important—you can see some reasons. Tell me more about that. Why do you say 5 instead of, say, 0 or 1?	*Reflection* *Follow-up question to elicit change talk*
PATIENT: Well, the nurse told me that exercise helps to decrease my insulin resistance.	*Change talk*
CLINICIAN: Yes, it does do that. What else?	
PATIENT: I guess it can help keep my weight down.	*Change talk*
CLINICIAN: And that's a good thing in managing diabetes. What else?	*Reflection—continuing the paragraph*
PATIENT: I don't know. My heart, maybe?	*Change talk*

CLINICIAN: Keeping your heart healthy and your blood pressure lower.

Reflection—continuing the paragraph

PATIENT: Right.

CLINICIAN: You'd like to hold on to your good health.

PATIENT: Yes.

Reflection

There are two more kinds of reflection that can be helpful when responding to sustain talk and reluctance. The first is termed an *amplified reflection*. When you hear sustain talk, you reflect it back and "turn up the volume" a bit on it. In other words, you restate it in even stronger terms than the patient did, and once again with absolutely no sarcasm. Doing this, we find, is even more likely to evoke change talk in the patient's next reply.

> *When you hear sustain talk, you reflect it back and "turn up the volume" a bit on it.*

PATIENT: I don't want to consider going on insulin.

CLINICIAN: There's no way you would ever do that.

Amplified reflection

PATIENT: Well, I think I will probably need insulin at some point.

Change talk

CLINICIAN: So, you just don't want to think about it right now, until it gets to the point that you need it to stay healthy and avoid complications.

Reflection

PATIENT: Right. Do you think I need it?

PATIENT: I don't want to give up being able to eat what I like.

CLINICIAN: No matter what the consequences are. It's that important to you to be able to eat whatever you like.

Continuing the paragraph with an amplified reflection

PATIENT: Well, I know I do need to make some changes.

Change talk

CLINICIAN: What changes do you think you might make?

Open question, asking for elaboration

Then there is the *double-sided reflection*, which includes both sustain talk and change talk that you have heard. This kind of reflection essentially acknowledges the patient's ambivalence.

PATIENT: Smoking is just a way to relax for me. I know it's not good for my health in the long run, but I've never tried to quit.

CLINICIAN: So, one part of you really enjoys smoking, and another part knows what it's doing to you.   *Double-sided reflection*

PATIENT: It's bad for my circulation, isn't it?   *Change talk*

CLINICIAN: Yes, and as you know that's a particular concern in diabetes. What else?

PATIENT: My heart, I guess—like blood pressure and heart attack.   *Change talk*

CLINICIAN: Right. On the one hand, you're used to smoking and it seems to relax you, and on the other hand you're well aware of how it can threaten your health and your life, particularly as a person with diabetes. That's a tough dilemma.   *Double-sided reflection*

PATIENT: I don't know if I really want to quit.   *Sustain talk*

CLINICIAN: Smoking might be so important to you that you need to keep on doing it no matter what the consequences are.   *Amplified reflection*

PATIENT: No—it's not *that* important.   *Change talk*

Notice two artful aspects of double-sided reflections. Most people tend to put *but* in the middle of their ambivalence: "I know it's bad for me, *but* I really enjoy it." The word "but" is a kind of eraser that discounts what went before it. In a double-sided reflection we try instead to put "and" in the middle (as illustrated above), emphasizing the both/and nature of ambivalence. Another useful tip is to put the sustain talk first and the change talk last when forming a double-sided reflection, because people are more likely to focus on what you said last (even without "but" in the middle). Consider what the patient in the example above might have said next if the clinician had instead given these double-sided reflections: "So one part of you knows what smoking is doing to you, but another part really enjoys it," or, "On the one hand, you're aware of how smoking can threaten your health and your life, but on the other hand you're used to smoking and it relaxes you." The double whammy of placing "but" in the middle and putting sustain talk last just seems to pull for more sustain talk.

This illustrates how in MI, once you get the hang of it, you're always thinking one step ahead: "If I say this, what is my patient likely to say next?" You consciously choose how you will respond—with the intention of evoking and strengthening your patients' own change talk so that they literally talk themselves into making healthy changes. You are not installing anything. The motivations for change are already there within the patient, and your task is to find and call them forth.

The Diabetes Educator: An Extended Example

Diabetes educators have a tough task. In a relatively short time you hope to provide patients with critical information needed to manage their diabetes well and persuade them to act on it. There is so much to cover, and you must decide what is most important to convey in the time allotted. Sometimes patients are still shocked by their new diagnosis of diabetes, or their eyes glaze over in reaction to all the new information they are receiving, but you hope that at least some of the information gets through to them.

Here is an example dialogue incorporating skills presented so far in this book. The patient is one whom you have seen before for diabetes education and who is here for a follow-up visit on referral from the primary care practitioner.

CLINICIAN: I see that your doctor asked you to come back and see me. Tell me how you've been doing since we met last.   *Open question*

PATIENT: My doctor thinks I could be trying harder to manage my diabetes.

CLINICIAN: And what do you think?   *Open question*

PATIENT: I probably could be doing more than I am. It's just that my life is so full with my job and family that I tend to put my own health on the back burner.   *Change talk and ambivalence*

CLINICIAN: It sounds like your life is pretty stressful, and also you know that you may be paying a price health-wise.

Double-sided reflection, with change talk last

PATIENT: I know it's dumb to be neglecting my own health, but I just feel like I'm doing the best I can right now.

Change talk + sustain talk = ambivalence

CLINICIAN: It may be that, given everything on your plate, you're already doing as much as you can to be healthy—and also here you are!

Double-sided reflection

PATIENT: I thought we could talk about it.

CLINICIAN: Definitely! I'm glad you came in even though your life is so busy.

Affirmation

PATIENT: I do want to see what I can do.

Change talk

CLINICIAN: Good! Well, there are quite a few things we could talk about today, and I don't want to overwhelm you with too much. So, help me decide what would be most useful for you. Here is a sheet with some possible topics we could discuss in relation to managing your diabetes and staying healthy. Have a look and let me know where we might start—or maybe there is something else you would prefer to discuss. That's why there is this bubble with a question mark. What do you think?

Introducing the bubble sheet (see Figure 3.1)

PATIENT: Exercise, maybe. I'm just not fitting it in, and I know that's not good.

Change talk

CLINICIAN: What do you know about how exercise helps?

Open question to evoke change talk

PATIENT: You explained to me last time about insulin resistance—that my body makes insulin but for some reason it's not working, and exercise can help that.

Change talk

CLINICIAN: Yes, that's right. You were really listening! Regular exercise does seem to help your body use the natural insulin you have.

Affirmation

PATIENT: But how much do I have to do?

CLINICIAN: Well, how much you can fit in is up to you. What most experts recommend now is about 150 minutes a week of moderate exercise.

Emphasizing personal choice

PATIENT: And what kind of exercise is that?

CLINICIAN: It can be whatever works for you—jogging, walking, going to the gym, bicycling, swimming—things that get your whole body moving. What kinds of exercise do you enjoy?

Emphasizing personal choice
Open question

PATIENT: Well, that's just the problem, though I do like how I feel after I've gone for a run sometimes.

Change talk

CLINICIAN: And how is that?

Open question, asking for elaboration of change talk

PATIENT: Sometimes I feel exhausted when I start out, but by the time I'm done I feel good—like tingling—and somehow I have more energy.

Change talk

CLINICIAN: It energizes you.

Reflection

PATIENT: Yes. And I feel good about having done it.

Change talk

CLINICIAN: About taking care of yourself.

Reflection

PATIENT: Yes. Now, the problem is time. I can't take off in the morning with the kids at home. I get them ready for school and then I go to work. When I get home I start thinking about dinner and get them started on their homework, and by the time they're ready for bed so am I.

Sustain talk

CLINICIAN: So, there really is just no space anywhere for you to fit in any exercise.

Amplified reflection

PATIENT: I do have an hour or so after they've gone to bed, but I can't leave the house then.

Change talk, but . . .

CLINICIAN: And that's when you feel exhausted.

Linking reflection

PATIENT: Right.

CLINICIAN: So, the challenge is how you could fit in some exercise without having to leave the kids alone. How might you do that?

Definite temptation to offer solutions, but the provider stays with an open question

PATIENT: I guess I could get a neighbor or sitter to stay there sometimes while I go for a run. Or I've thought about getting a machine at home—an elliptical or treadmill or something like that . . .

Change talk

CLINICIAN: That would mean you don't have to leave the house. How possible is that for you?

Reflection and closed question

PATIENT: I've seen them on sale, and I have some room in the back of the house.

Change talk

CLINICIAN: Well, it sounds like you have some good ideas there. You already know how helpful exercise can be with insulin resistance, and you enjoy it when you do fit it in. We haven't talked about weekends, but even on workdays you said you could get someone to come over while the kids are in bed to let you go for a run. You also could get some exercise equipment to have at home so you don't have to go out. Those seem like ideas that could work for you.

Affirmation

Summary

PATIENT: I think so.

Change talk

CLINICIAN: So, what do you think you'll do?

Open question to elicit mobilizing change talk

PATIENT: I'm going to look for a sale and get something I like that will let me exercise at home.

Change talk (commitment)

CLINICIAN: Good! I look forward to hearing about that. Now, what else is there on this sheet that you might like to discuss today?

More evoking

PATIENT: Well, I do have some questions about medications . . .

Key Points

- People can and do literally talk themselves into (or out of) change.

- Particular types of speech—change talk and sustain talk—signal a person's movement toward or away from change.

- A key first skill is to recognize change talk when you hear it and know that it is particularly important.

- The balance between change talk and sustain talk predicts the likelihood that change will occur.

- Particular interviewing skills can be used to evoke and respond to change talk.

- The balance of change talk matters, and is highly responsive to the clinician's MI skills.

- Change talk represents immediate feedback from the patient that you're doing something right.

CHAPTER 6

Offering Information
and Advice

As a diabetes professional, you do have important expertise to share with patients, and they count on you to do so. Most often this takes the form of conveying information about diabetes and offering advice on diabetes management. For licensed prescribers and pharmacists this also includes the monitoring of medications (see Chapters 9 and 11).

When what is needed is lifestyle behavior change, though, a one-way transmission of information and advice is usually insufficient. As discussed in Chapter 2, the patient's own expertise and collaboration are needed. Striking a balance can be particularly challenging during early consultations, where you may feel the need to convey a lot of information in a relatively short period of time.

We begin with two general guidelines about dispensing information and advice:

1. Offer only what is needed and likely to be used, and
2. Do so only with the patient's permission.

Necessary and Sufficient

A common error in diabetes care is to offer too much information and advice at one time. Often patients need less information than one might think. Diabetes is a chronic condition to be managed over time, and patients vary in their tolerance for advice and new information. What is truly *necessary* to convey in a patient's first visit? Given the patient's condition

> *A common error in diabetes care is to offer too much information and advice at one time.*

and capacities, what is most likely to be *useful*? This is the art of conveying what is necessary and sufficient.

Imagine you are learning a complex medical procedure to which you have just been introduced. You listen and watch and then try your hand at it for the first time with supervision. If your supervisor next tells you 17 things to do differently next time, what is the likely outcome? You might be able to remember and implement a few of his or her instructions, but the volume of input can be overwhelming and disheartening. A good teacher will help you step by step to make improvements in practice, sometimes one component at a time.

It's the same with patients. What is *most important* to focus on first? What change is going to be easiest to implement and most likely to make a significant difference? What change seems most acceptable and possible from the patient's perspective? What is the next step, and what does the patient want and need to know in order to take that step?

Too often overlooked is what patients *do* know. It is redundant, even insulting, to tell people what they already know. An early study of MI in prenatal clinics focused on women who were drinking alcohol while pregnant (Handmaker, Miller, & Manicke, 1999). The righting reflex was salient: to lecture these women about the dangers of alcohol to the unborn child. Wasn't it, after all, our urgent professional responsibility to do so? Instead, we decided to ask them, "What do you already know about the effects of alcohol on an unborn child?" The women already knew about 90% of what we were about to tell them, and in this situation it was the *patients telling us* (rather than vice versa) why they should not be drinking during pregnancy (in other words, change talk). For the remaining 10%, we could fill in missing information or correct their misunderstandings. That meant it was necessary and sufficient to say only 10% of what we had planned in most cases, with the added benefit of women telling themselves why they needed to make a change.

Three Kinds of Permission

Besides offering only what is necessary and sufficient, it is also wise to have your patient's permission. In MI, we describe three ways to have permission to offer information or advice. The first and simplest is when your patients ask for it:

"What can I do to decrease my A1c level?"
"Do you think I should be taking medication for this?"
"What does depression have to do with diabetes?"
"What do you think I should do?"

Questions like these are an invitation to provide some of what you know—not *everything* you know, but we'll come back to that.

A second way to have permission is for you to ask for it. Our experience is that when we ask permission to give information or advice, 99% of the time patients grant it.

> "I have one concern about your plan. Is it OK if I share it with you?"
> "I wonder if it would be helpful for me to describe some things that other patients have done successfully in this situation."
> "May I make a suggestion?"

There is something about asking permission that seems to lower the barriers to communication and make it more likely the patient will listen to what you have to say. Asking permission is an act of collaboration, reflecting a respectful partnership between practitioner and client.

But what about a clinical situation where it seems disingenuous to ask for permission because you're going to tell the patient regardless, perhaps because you perceive it to be a duty of your profession? If you asked for permission and the patient said "No," you would still feel obligated to say it. Here we suggest the third option of qualifying what you are about to say, particularly by acknowledging and honoring the patient's autonomy. This isn't quite asking for permission, but it does give patients implicit permission to disregard what you are about to say. Letting patients know that they don't have to listen to you (which, of course, they don't) makes it more likely they will hear you. You are not granting them anything they didn't already have. Some examples:

> "This may or may not interest or concern you . . . "
> "I don't know if this will make any sense to you . . . "
> "You may not agree—and that's fine—but I want you to know . . . "

Manageable Doses

Another guideline is to offer information or advice in digestible bite-sized pieces. You may have a lot of ground to cover, but you don't have to do it all in one long speech. Within what is necessary and sufficient, think manageable chunks.

This couples with another recommendation, namely, to surround these chunks of information with close listening. A mnemonic here is "elicit–provide–elicit" (E-P-E). Start off by asking what the patient wants to know or already knows, or ask permission, or ask what would be

Start off by asking what the patient wants to know or already knows.

helpful. Then provide a manageable dose of information or advice, followed by eliciting the patient's perspective once again:

"What do you think about that?"
"Does that make sense to you?"
"Was that clear enough? Any questions?"
"Now tell me your take on this."
"What else would you like to know?"

A large amount of information can be conveyed in this E-P-E-P-E sequence, particularly if you first learn and set aside what the patient already knows. E-P-E creates the kind of two-way flow of information that is needed for negotiating lifestyle and behavior change.

Give Patients a Choice

Most people prefer having options from which to choose rather than being limited to one possibility. When there are alternatives, present them:

"Of these topics, what would be most helpful to discuss today?"
"There are a number of things that can help to manage your diabetes . . ."
"Of these three options, which one sounds best to you?"
"What is your hunch about what would work best for you?"

Presenting multiple options also helps to avoid a trap that is easy to fall into when you present just one option at a time:

CLINICIAN: There are some medications that can be helpful when you're depressed.

PATIENT: I don't like to take medications. I can do this on my own.

CLINICIAN: Oh, well, we have a support group here at the clinic for . . .

PATIENT: I'm just not very comfortable talking in groups.

CLINICIAN: OK. Let me tell you, then, about a treatment called cognitive-behavioral therapy. It helps examine your thought patterns and how they influence your mood.

PATIENT: Are you saying it's all in my head?

You see the problem. You present one possibility, and the patient tells you what's wrong with it. Suddenly you find yourself in exactly the wrong chair, arguing for change while the patient argues against it. A different approach is to ask the patient to choose among options.

CLINICIAN: I agree, depression and diabetes is a bad combination; so, let me describe some of the options that are available to help prevent and alleviate depression, whether or not people have diabetes. I'll mention them briefly and then ask you about your hunches— which one or two sound like they might work best for you.

The mental task here is to choose rather than to refute, and people are more likely to accept and stick with that which they have freely chosen. It helps people to, first, find and then own the solutions for the issue being discussed.

Glucose Monitoring: Offering Information and Advice

To illustrate the processes described in this chapter, here is a sample conversation from a consultation in which a person recently diagnosed with T2D diabetes is being introduced to the use of a glucose monitor. There is information to be conveyed, and the clinician obviously hopes to encourage the patient to use the monitor regularly. Nevertheless, the spirit and style of the interview is distinctly MI. The clinician is watching for change talk about diabetes control in general and about self-monitoring in particular.

CLINICIAN: We've been discussing how glucose and insulin work in your body. Would it be all right now if we talked a bit about monitoring your blood glucose? That's one important tool in managing your diabetes. | *Asking permission*

PATIENT: Sure. OK.

CLINICIAN: Let me ask you first what you already know about why it's important to track your blood levels and how to do it. I don't want to tell you things that you already know. | *Elicit*

PATIENT: I guess the goal is to keep my blood sugar level low so that this will help me know where I am.

CLINICIAN: Good—yes. Not too low, but just right. Monitoring is a way to know where your glucose level is at any given time, and there are other | *Affirmation*

benefits, too. So, what do you know about why it's important to keep your glucose tightly controlled?	*Elicit*

PATIENT: It can go too high or too low, and both are unhealthy?

CLINICIAN: That's right. In fact, it can be dangerous if your level gets too far out of bounds.	*Provide*

PATIENT: And what are the bounds?	*Giving permission to offer information*

CLINICIAN: The normal range when fasting, like first thing in the morning, is 80 to 120, and for people with diabetes we like to see it between 80 on the low side and 180 2 hours after meals. Does that make sense to you?	*Provide* *Elicit*

PATIENT: Yes. I remember that my morning level was 127 on my last checkup, and that's why the doctor did some additional tests.

CLINICIAN: Right. That's above normal levels, and she did the right thing to follow up with the hemoglobin A1c test. What do you know about that test?	*Provide* *Elicit*

PATIENT: Not much. She said it's like an average sugar level over a longer time.

CLINICIAN: It is. I can explain more about how it works, if you like, but basically it reflects your average sugar level over the past 3 months, and so it's also a pretty good indicator of how well you are managing your diabetes. Do you remember what your A1c value was?	*Provide* *Elicit*

PATIENT: I think it was 7.4, and she said that means I have diabetes and I should come see you.

CLINICIAN: Right. So she wants us to talk   *Provide*
about what you can do to manage
your diabetes, and one of those is
to check your sugar levels regularly.
What's your feeling about that?   *Elicit*

PATIENT: I guess if I need to do it I need   *Change talk*
to do it.

CLINICIAN: Good. So, let's talk about   *Renewing permission*
how you do it if that's OK. Have you
ever seen or used one of these? (*Takes*   *Elicit*
out a glucose monitor.)

PATIENT: No. I've heard about them. You
stick your finger, right?

CLINICIAN: That's right, with a lancet.   *Provide*
They keep making these better. This
lancing device has a spring in it that
you click back like this (*demon-*
strates), place it against your finger-
tip, and release it with this button
here (*demonstrates*). Want to try   *Elicit*
that?—without sticking your finger
first.

PATIENT: OK. (*Tries it.*) I didn't see anything.

CLINICIAN: The lancet is really small and   *Provide*
fast, and it doesn't come out very
far. You can also adjust it here to
change how far it comes out. Keep
the setting low enough to just get a
small droplet of blood—and you may
hardly feel the stick.

PATIENT: Can it be used more than once?   *Requesting information*

CLINICIAN: Yes, it can. You can change it   *Provide*
to a new lancet every time, which is
another way to avoid pain if it bothers you, but some of my patients use
the same lancet a number of times.
It's up to you how often you want to   *Emphasizing personal*
change it, but if it starts to hurt, then   *choice*
you rotate this until it clicks once
(*demonstrates*) and you have a brand

new lancet. Now, there's one thing   *Type 3 permission*
I need to tell you here that is very
important, and I'll be curious if it
makes sense to you.

PATIENT: Oh, what's that?

CLINICIAN: No one else besides you   *Provide*
should ever use this. Don't let anyone
else try it out. Even a tiny amount of
blood can get onto this lance, so it's
strictly a one-person instrument. Can   *Elicit*
you see why?

PATIENT: So you don't get somebody else's
blood, a serious disease of some kind.

CLINICIAN: Exactly. That's why you never   *Provide*
share it with anyone else, even if
you've just changed to a new lance.
OK?   *Elicit*

PATIENT: OK. I understand.

CLINICIAN: Now, can I show you one   *Asking permission*
more trick before you try it out?

PATIENT: OK. I understand so far.

CLINICIAN: Put your hands together like   *Provide*
this (*demonstrates*), as someone
might do if they were praying. The
side surface that you can see now is
the best place on your fingers to use
the lancing device. Avoid your finger-
tips that have a lot of nerve endings,
and also stay away from bone. Right
here along the side is the best place to
test. Any questions about that?   *Elicit*

PATIENT: So, the best place is on the side
here where it's soft.

CLINICIAN: Right—not on your finger-
tips, and not on these bony places.
OK? So, if you're willing, I'd like
you to try it out now with a finger of
your choosing. Ready to try it?   *Asking permission*

PATIENT: I guess so.

CLINICIAN: So, this little hole is where the lancet comes out. Hold that right up against the side of your finger. Just around to the side a little more, closer to your fingernail. Right after you click it turn your attention to pressing next to the stick point—just like this—so that a little drop of blood comes out. You don't need much of a drop with this model. I find if I focus right away on applying pressure, then I don't feel the stick so much. *Provide*

PATIENT: Do you have diabetes?

CLINICIAN: Yes, I do. That's one reason I enjoy this work. *Provide*
OK, so give it a try. Click the spring back—good—pick a finger—OK, your ring finger—and gently press it against the side of your finger—that's good. Now click . . . and press to get a small drop. Good! That's enough. How was that? *Affirmation*

Elicit

PATIENT: OK. Not too bad.

CLINICIAN: Now I'm going to put a test strip in the meter here like this, and just touch the end of it to that drop of blood. There. And in a few seconds it will give us a reading: 178.

PATIENT: That's pretty high?

CLINICIAN: Well, after you've eaten it's normal for blood sugar to go up, especially when you have diabetes. A good goal is to keep the peaks under 180—so, it's just below that. You can use these tests to figure out how much particular foods drive your sugar level up, because it's different for different people. I recommend that you test your blood 2 hours after eating and learn how different foods affect you. Does that make sense? *Provide*

Elicit

PATIENT: So, I should test after every meal?

CLINICIAN: With type 2 diabetes, just twice a day should be enough. You can test at different times on different days—before you eat anything in the morning, or 2 hours after a meal. You can also try before and after exercise to see how that affects your sugar. Keep records of all the readings for a while—they will be on the meter's memory, too, but write down the time of day and whether you're fasting or when you ate. Does that sound realistic for you?   *Provide*

                                                                    Elicit

PATIENT: Yes, it doesn't take very long. I just have to remember to do it.   *Change talk*

CLINICIAN: Great. Now, when is your next check-up with your doctor?   *Closed question*

PATIENT: In about 2 months.

CLINICIAN: OK, good. So keep good records of your blood test results, time of tests and meals, and then take that in to your doctor. She can compare it with your next A1c test.   *Provide*

PATIENT: To check up on me.

CLINICIAN: To see how you're doing and what a next step would be. And in the meantime you'll be learning a lot about how different foods and exercise affect your blood sugar. Think of it as being a personal scientist—observing and learning how your body works. Are you willing to do that?   *Closed question asking for mobilizing change talk*

PATIENT: Sure.   *Change talk*

CLINICIAN: What other questions do you have about monitoring your glucose level?   *Elicit*

PATIENT: I heard you can also test other places, like on your hand or arm.

CLINICIAN: There are meters that do
     that, but the levels are different, and
     I recommend that you start out with   *Provide*
     this one for your fingers. This meter
     is yours, and here's a small supply of
     test strips and a form for recording
     your readings. With a prescription
     you can get more at a pharmacy.
     Anything else about glucose testing?   *Elicit*

PATIENT: No, I think I can do it. I have   *Change talk*
     the prescription for test strips.

CLINICIAN: All right. And there are
     instructions there in the box as well.
     Now, can we take a few minutes   *Asking permission*
     more to talk about carbohydrates, or
     is that about enough information for
     one day?

As an example of an early visit (where so much is new for the patient), the clinician here is providing a lot of information and advice, and thus the OARS skills are less prevalent. Even so, the process is collaborative, and the clinician does not present very much information without checking in to elicit the patient's responses. It's a very different style from just down-loading lots of new information and assuming that the patient understands.

Key Points

- Providing information and advice is seldom enough when what is needed is lifestyle behavior change.
- Offer information and advice only with the patient's permission.
- Avoid telling patients what they already know.
- Decide what information is necessary and sufficient.
- Offer information in small manageable chunks, using the elicit–provide–elicit sequence.

PART II

MOTIVATIONAL INTERVIEWING AND COMMON CHALLENGES IN DIABETES CARE

CHAPTER 7

A New Diagnosis of Diabetes

People often feel emotionally overwhelmed when they find out they have diabetes. There is so much new information to take in, and the challenges of self-care can be formidable, reflecting major changes in physical activity, adopting a healthy diet (often with caloric and content restrictions), initiation of blood glucose testing and responses to test results; taking numerous medications (often at multiple times a day); managing psychological stress while hoping to be able to avoid the elevated blood glucose levels associated with it; preventive measures to avoid foot ulcers; regular eye exams and dental care; and developing a plan for managing diabetes in the context of acute illnesses. To make matters even worse, some people are diagnosed with T2D in the context of other threatening conditions, such as an acute myocardial infarction (heart attack) (Tenerz et al., 2003) or diabetic retinopathy.

One common and understandable response to all of this is avoidance: flight instead of fight. This avoidance can look like denial *("It's better not to know")* or fatalism ("There's nothing I can do about it anyhow").

"Maybe I don't really have diabetes."

"It's just too much to think about."

"I don't have a long enough day to do all of this diabetes stuff."

"It's easier for me to eat what I want if I don't test my blood glucose."

"What will be will be."

"When your time comes up, there's nothing you can do about it."

"If I go back, the doctor will just tell me about more things I need to do."

"I saw a nice diabetes educator, but I feel overwhelmed with all that information."

A primary task during the first year after the diagnosis of diabetes is helping people choose fight rather than flight by taking an active role in maintaining and improving their own health instead of shutting down and tuning out. The collaborative and accepting spirit of MI provides an important foundation for supporting active self-care. This chapter will illustrate how the clinical skills of MI described in preceding chapters can be useful when a patient faces newly diagnosed diabetes.

We will use a case example to illustrate how MI can be used for patients with newly diagnosed diabetes. The person at the center of this chapter is Frank, a 58-year-old businessman who was recently diagnosed with diabetes during a hospitalization for an acute myocardial infarction. The undiagnosed diabetes was likely long-standing. He has a strong family history of T2D. He has smoked cigarettes for 35 years. Before this cardiac event occurred he took no medications; he left the hospital with a list of six medications. While in the hospital he was seen by diabetes educators, a dietitian, and a nurse. The dietitian shared information with him about

---

I was medically naïve and in my third year of college at age 20 when I was diagnosed with T1D. Except for an aunt with Parkinson's disease, I was unfamiliar with serious chronic health conditions. My diabetic ketoacidosis was so mild it's unlikely I would be admitted today. However, in the early 1970s I ended up in the hospital (without an IV) and spent 5 days learning how to give myself insulin, along with education that focused on how my life would need to change.

The hospitalization brought my enormous medical naiveté to an abrupt end. During those 5 days I got to know my diabetes well. But I ended up with lots more questions than answers when I went home. To me it was an upsetting oddity that elevated blood glucose levels could cause eye disease and blindness, end-stage kidney disease, heart attacks, nerve injuries, and foot ulcers leading to lower limb amputations. My main feeling was an incredulous numbness. Several times during that hospitalization I thought scaring me about complications was a ruse to scare me into taking insulin, something I actually wanted to do. It beat the option of dying!

After leaving the hospital, my great concern was dying prematurely. Although I knew I was not immortal, at that age I could still think and at times act as though there was no such thing as dying. Diabetes ended that fantasy. I resolved to do whatever was needed so that I could live each day and hopefully for a few more years. But I also struggled internally on rare occasions when health care providers I saw did not seem to understand what I found difficult about *my diabetes*. That ultimately led me to work on the skills needed to help people struggling with chronic conditions. And it launched a trajectory that led me to MI.

—MPS

I was 60 when my doctor noticed a high fasting glucose and, on subsequent testing, an elevated A1c. "We could say you have diabetes or call it prediabetes, but either way it's time to talk about making some changes."

I was stunned. It had never occurred to me that I would develop diabetes. I was not overweight and ate a fairly healthy diet. I had been lax about physical activity, but otherwise I had few risk factors except choosing the wrong grandparents. My grandmother was diagnosed with diabetes at age 60, and my sister died in childhood from complications of T1D.

My immediate question was "What do I need to do to stay healthy?" I went to see a diabetes educator who showed me how to test my blood and gave me a 1-hour download of how-to information complete with plastic food portions. More helpful to me was a savvy book, *The First Year: Type 2 Diabetes: An Essential Guide for the Newly Diagnosed*, by Gretchen Becker, herself a person living with diabetes, which offered a patient, step-by-step approach with practical options and useful perspectives. I am a scientist, and one idea that definitely stuck with me was using blood testing to discover how specific foods affect my own glucose level. Through experimentation I learned to avoid particular foods that might have seemed innocuous (like popcorn and watermelon). I still use regular testing to keep from kidding myself.

—WRM

healthy eating. The nurse discussed the importance of follow-up health care visits and regular self-examination of his feet. She also showed him how to check his blood glucose levels, something he is doing twice daily now. His discharge plan included appointments with a dietitian, his primary care physician, and the cardiologist who treated his heart attack. We will see parts of two appointments during his first year with diabetes, one with his usual physician and one with his dietitian.

Engaging

The initial MI process of engaging is a foundation for working effectively with people, but when people know that their lifestyle involves unhealthy behaviors such as smoking, they may avoid talking about it. Often smokers are frustrated by past admonitions about smoking from health care providers and indeed by many coworkers, family members, or friends. Especially in the health care setting, this may limit the willingness of people who smoke to spontaneously share information about their tobacco habit.

Frank's first appointment following his myocardial infarction was with his usual physician. At his hospital discharge he was told not to smoke. However, the nurse who escorted him to the consultation room and updated his recent history told the doctor she could smell cigarette smoke on the patient. She was frustrated by Frank, who spoke freely about wanting to avoid another heart attack. She did not offer Frank any advice. Instead, she said to his physician, "I don't understand how anyone could continue smoking after almost dying of a heart attack." She also told the doctor that Frank would benefit from a serious conversation about the dangers of diabetes and smoking.

The nurse's concern aligned with the fact that cardiovascular risks increase significantly for people with diabetes who smoke. Diabetes and smoking are independent variables that increase the risks for heart attacks. The risk of a heart attack for people with T2D is two to four times higher than in people without diabetes. Smoking further increases heart attack risk, making it 1.7 times more likely in people with T2D (AHA Scientific Statement, 2013). So, people with T2D who smoke have a 3.7- to 5.7-fold increase in the risk of a heart attack when compared to nonsmokers without T2D. MI provides a collaborative approach for working with people in this risky area of diabetes care.

An Interview with a Physician

The physician welcomed Frank in a relaxed, friendly way. She told him she had been looking forward to seeing him ever since the cardiologist had informed her of his recent hospitalization. She listened attentively as he answered her question about how he was feeling. In addition to no cardiac symptoms, he told her he is appropriately taking six medications, testing his blood glucose levels twice daily, and participating in a cardiac rehabilitation program. He expressed frustration about having diabetes but also said he is willing to do what it takes to care for it. However, he then quickly qualified his willingness: "I have to find the time to be able to do all of this." He also wanted to return to work the following week.

PHYSICIAN: You're working on a lot of new tasks. You are doing well with medications, glucose testing, and cardiac rehab. You're eager to get back to work, too. You are facing this situation well. What is this like for you?

FRANK: It's a bit overwhelming. I not only have to eat differently, I have to eat less. That's not easy for me to do. The blood glucose tests have shown me how my eating affects my diabetes. It's mostly bad news—my levels are higher than the goal they wanted

The physician provides affirmations about Frank's self-care and desire to get back to work. She then asks an open question about other areas of his self-care.

me to have in the morning, 90–120. They also said it should be less than 180 2 hours after a meal. But my results are higher than that. Maybe there's a problem with the medicine. Most of the pills I take are for my heart. Metformin is the only thing I'm taking for diabetes.

PHYSICIAN: You'd want to achieve lower levels when you test your blood glucose. The downloaded results from your glucose meter are a bit high, but the levels are not really that problematic.

After a reflection the physician provides information to Frank by appropriately reassuring him that his blood glucose values will improve.

FRANK: Will they come down?

PHYSICIAN: At the hospital they gave you a schedule for increasing your metformin dose. The levels should improve as you get to the target dose in a few days. I'm wondering if your concern about glucose levels might be related to something challenging about the dietary changes recommended to you when you met with the hospital dietitian.

The physician answers Frank's question and makes a reflection that "guesses" that Frank is challenged with all the dietary changes he is facing.

FRANK: Wait a minute! I used to eat all of a large container of ice cream for dessert several nights a week when I watched TV in the evening. I am no longer doing that. In fact, all I'm eating for dessert now is a serving of fruit—and nothing when I'm watching TV. But I don't like not being able to eat steak and fries as much as I want to. When I'm traveling with my job, I look forward to that kind of food. Just looking at my size lets you know I enjoy eating. I'm dealing with the double whammy—diabetes and a heart attack! It would be nice to be successful with all this stuff. But it's going to be hard to do. I've worked hard all my life, and I know how to

Frank promptly corrects her reflection. A valuable part of MI is the instant feedback patients give to practitioners. The reflection was promptly corrected with the mobilizing change talk Frank used to describe the alterations he has already made in his dinner and after-dinner eating habits.

get things done. I've already changed some of the ways I'm eating.

PHYSICIAN: Good for you! You developed your own plan to significantly lower the calories and fat in your desserts at dinnertime. Desserts and snacking like you were doing with ice cream are hard habits to change. But you're doing that now. There are also concerns about giving up what you like to eat. Those concerns are especially important with the travel you do with your job. You will be eating in restaurants more. You're working hard to accomplish your diabetes goals. You are also thoughtful about your blood glucose levels.

The physician uses a positive, affirming approach with Frank. She affirms the work he has done. This differs from reminding Frank of the complications of diabetes and then providing a list of needed behaviors to avoid them. The affirmations are not a form of "cheerleading." The physician listens actively to affirm Frank's strengths.

FRANK: What you said sounds right. I also think you understand how hard all of this stuff is. I'm going to see the dietitian again next week.

Frank continues with change talk in his mention of seeing the dietitian.

PHYSICIAN: Would it be OK with you if we talked about smoking?

The physician returns to the focusing process. She wants to widen the topics included in this visit by asking Frank's permission to bring up a sensitive topic. Asking permission respects his autonomy. People usually agree to conversations when their permission is sought.

FRANK: I was hoping to get out of here without talking about cigarettes. We've talked about it in the past, and I'll go along with this. But I have to tell you something really important first. I have never been in a situation as bad as this. It's pretty stressful for me right now. I haven't been able to work, and my income has taken a big hit. I've just survived something that could've killed me, and I'm trying to

Although Frank grants permission for the conversation, he responds to the smoking topic with copious sustain talk.

deal with something that doesn't go away—diabetes. Cigarettes help me with these stresses.

PHYSICIAN: It's hard for you to imagine how you could handle the stress in your life right now without smoking. It's that important to you.

The physician continues reflective listening with another reflection.

FRANK: I know I need to quit, but I'm just not ready at this point.

Change talk and sustain talk

PHYSICIAN: You do understand how risky it is for you to keep smoking now, and whenever you're willing we can discuss how you might quit. So, if quitting smoking is not an option now, I wonder if there is some other change you might make in the meantime to get your diabetes under better control.

The interviewer reflects the change talk and keeps the door open while moving on to something that is more feasible for today.

FRANK: I'm going to see the dietitian next week for some ideas about eating healthy when I travel.

PHYSICIAN: Yes, good. That can make a difference. You've already made some good changes. What else do you think might help you get your glucose down?

Again, the physician responds with an affirmation followed by an open question.

FRANK: They told me that I should exercise more.

PHYSICIAN: What do you think about that? Does it seem possible? What small changes might you make?

FRANK: I could take the stairs instead of the elevator. (Laughs)

Frank ventures forward with some change talk.

PHYSICIAN: Actually that's a very good example—a small change that fits into your regular routine. What else?

FRANK: My wife and I are trying out a water aerobics class.

PHYSICIAN: You think you will be able to do more as the acute stage of this ends and you get back to your usual routines.

The physician responds selectively to the patient's perspective that his work routine may offer him an opportunity to reorganize his life.

FRANK: Having had this heart attack and then finding out about diabetes are things I don't need. I feel stuck with this stuff now. But I am willing to keep working on it.

Despite his frustrations, Frank uses preparatory change talk about his willingness to provide self-care.

PHYSICIAN: So, let's see if I understand where you are right now. You have a plan to address your eating at restaurants and talk with the dietitian. We also discussed the healthy changes you've made at your evening meals and your awareness and concerns about your blood glucose levels. Even though these changes are difficult, you are sticking with them. Am I on target?

The physician creates a transition with a summary. She specifically plucks out change talk she has heard Frank use during the encounter. The importance placed on change talk is related to the fact that the more change talk someone uses the more likely he or she is to change (Magill, Apodaca, Barnett, & Mobti, 2010).

FRANK: Yes, you are.

PHYSICIAN: Are you comfortable with a follow-up appointment in 2 months?

The last statement is a closed question.

FRANK: I'll do that.

Reactance

Think of how often people seek health care and at the same time continue behaviors that actually undermine their health. To be sure, factors such as addictions, mental health conditions, cognitive problems, and poverty can be significant barriers to better health behavior.

Does Frank's situation seem like a behavioral paradox? True, he is addicted to nicotine and also suffered a heart attack and nearly died. Why would someone who faced death and survived continue to cling to cigarettes?

When people are told they have a serious problem, they also experience a loss of freedom. The global changes in the "things to do list" of diabetes or cardiac self-care are good examples of what can lead people to feel as though their freedoms are being crimped. This situation is called psychological reactance (Worchel, 2013). Whenever people experience a potential loss of freedom, there is a natural tendency to reassert it.

At the onset of diabetes, people often find it easier to adopt one or more new self-care behaviors than to change unhealthy behaviors they associate with past comforts. Frank copiously used change talk in the interview. He talked about wanting to care for his diabetes and is actually doing a good job with those tasks. He also wants to avoid another cardiac event. He even acknowledged that he will have to stop using tobacco "sometime." But, for now, he is holding on to his freedom to smoke as he deals with the overwhelming changes in his life and as he begins the tasks of self-care for his diabetes.

> At the onset of diabetes, people often find it easier to adopt one or more new self-care behaviors than to change unhealthy behaviors they associate with past comforts.

A temptation when you hear reactance is to follow with the righting reflex and push against it, which usually makes matters worse. The physician using MI with Frank briefly explored smoking and then guided the conversation toward other areas. Rather than confronting him, she intentionally avoided discord and controversy, leaving the door open for future opportunities to discuss tobacco use. Returning to a collaborative conversation is more valuable than patient dissatisfaction and a decision not to return for future appointments or disengagement from future discussions of tobacco. Follow-up is the necessary ingredient for helping people as they develop self-care plans. Frank indicated he wants to continue working on diabetes self-care. He also responded agreeably to a return visit.

Chapter 12 offers additional examples of using MI to address tobacco addiction and other areas of substance use.

An Interview with a Dietitian

The subject of food and dietary restriction is likely to evoke reactance, the perceived loss of freedom to have favorite foods and enjoyable meals with friends and family. This is an area where a collaborative (rather than prescriptive) approach is particularly important. The task is to figure out how patients can fit the needed changes into their cultural and social circumstances while retaining the joy of eating and shared meals (Vanstone et al., 2013). It's a challenging task and one that definitely benefits from patients' own expertise about themselves.

The following interview illustrates how MI can be used to guide conversations toward exploring healthy eating choices. Frank focuses his concern on eating in restaurants. He believes this will damage his current progress with weight loss. The dietitian helps him to reframe his thoughts about the challenges of eating in restaurants. Evoking and responding selectively to change talk help him develop a new perspective for an area that challenges him.

Frank, accompanied by his wife, is seeing the same dietitian he saw in the hospital. The dietitian had asked Frank to be sure his wife, Brenda, accompanied him on this visit and added, "When one person in a family has diabetes, the whole family has diabetes." He warmly welcomes them as he weighs Frank.

DIETITIAN: It's been 3 weeks since I last saw the two of you when Frank was in the hospital. You've done well with weight loss during that time, Frank. Your weight is down 4%— you dropped from 242 pounds to 232 pounds since you went home from the hospital. Your BMI [body mass index], a measurement based on your weight and height, has dropped over 1 point, from 34.6 to 33.3. How did you do that?

The dietitian begins with an affirmation about Frank's weight loss. Affirmations strengthen the process of engaging.

BRENDA: Frank is eating much differently. He's not eating large bowls of ice cream or handfuls of cookies for dessert. And we've started a water aerobics program three times a week.

Frank has made significant changes in the self-care of his diabetes although he still smokes.

FRANK: Brenda and I are talking more about health than about food. The water aerobics has been good for me. And Brenda has done all the food work. She's actually helped me a lot to get the ideas you discussed with us into action. But I'm worried. I've gone back to work, and I will soon be traveling out of town for several days at a time. In the restaurants I used to go to, I didn't pick healthy foods. It may be harder to continue weight loss when I'm eating at restaurants.

After the dietitian briefly engages Frank, he outlines what he wants to focus on.

DIETITIAN: You spoke of that challenge in the hospital. Can you tell me more about it?

The interviewer responds with an open question.

FRANK: Restaurants often serve more food than I'm eating now and I'm not good at leaving things on my plate. You're not going to like this one either: I eat lunch at fast-food places. For dinner, I used to eat steak and potatoes frequently. You know, eating out involves lots of carbs—bread, rice, potatoes, or sometimes pasta. It's not like what I've been eating lately.

Frank describes the issues that concern him.

DIETITIAN: So, you've made a good head start with healthy eating at home, and now the challenge is how to do that when you're not home and are eating in restaurants. How do you think you might stay healthy when you're on the road?

The dietitian affirms Frank's initial progress, and rather than immediately offering suggestions he asks for Frank's own ideas.

FRANK: I want to use the swimming pools at hotels when I'm traveling. I won't be doing the same aerobic stuff we're doing in the classes, but I'll be walking and swimming in the water for 30 minutes in the evening before supper.

Frank uses change talk as he describes how he wants to continue his physical activity.

DIETITIAN: That's a great idea. You will be able to continue your physical activity. I also asked you to come in today Brenda, but it sounds like we will be talking more about food in restaurants instead of food at home.

BRENDA: That's OK. We also go out for dinner when he's home. I want to help him, and I also would like him to lose some weight.

DIETITIAN: You expressed some concern about fast-food restaurants. Would you like some ideas about eating in fast-food and other restaurants?

The interviewer asks for Frank's permission to provide information and advice about eating in restaurants.

FRANK: Sure.

DIETITIAN: The same approaches you use at home with portion size apply in fast-food and other restaurants. If you're tempted by the food, you can always ask to be served less than a full order. It sounds like you're already eating food based on portion-sized servings. Ask how big the servings are before you decide on how much you want. And in fast-food restaurants avoid the large-sized meals or large orders of french fries. Diet soda has no calories. Regular soda has a lot of sugar. I have booklets with the calories and grams of fat and carbs for each item in most fast-food restaurants. I will give them to you. You can also use a smartphone to look up those things. What do you think about these ideas?

Oops—way too much provide and not enough elicit! The routine (described in Chapter 6) is elicit–provide–elicit, usually with relatively small doses of providing information and advice. The expected result would be sustain talk.

FRANK: I understand what you're saying. I'd like to read the written material. I'm not sure it will help me when I'm by myself. It's harder for me to control how much I eat when I'm alone.

And, sure enough, Frank responds with some sustain talk.

DIETITIAN: You're concerned about eating too much, especially when you're on your own.

The dietitian responds to Frank's personal disclosure.

FRANK: I have always enjoyed eating. When I'm with my wife, it is easier to eat less. We sort of work on it together.

DIETITIAN: When you're together you help each other, so it really is when you're away from home that you need some new routines. What changes do you think might make the biggest difference when you're away?

Reflection

Open question—elicit

FRANK: I could choose healthier restaurants and stay away from fast-food places.

DIETITIAN: You're right about that. There aren't so many healthy choices in most fast-food places, so avoiding them is one good option. What else?

Provide

Elicit

FRANK: I know you're right about sodas. They're loaded with sugar. I don't really like the taste of diet sodas, but I could probably get used to them or have something else, like unsweetened tea.

DIETITIAN: That one change can make a real difference in your glucose levels. I don't know if you get the large-sized "big-gulp" sodas, but just one of those can have 600 or 700 calories in it, compared to 0. Is that a change that is realistic for you?

Provide

Elicit

FRANK: Yes, that's something I can do.

Change talk

DIETITIAN: That would be a good start. It's really a matter of making a series of small changes, and actually that's one that can make a big difference. Now let me ask you this: How important would you say it is, on a 0–10 scale, to eat in a more healthy way and get your diabetes under better control? If 0 means "not at all important" and 10 means "the most important thing in my life right now," what number would you give yourself?

Instead of providing more advice, the dietitian elects to use importance and confidence rulers (Miller & Rollnick, 2013, pp. 174–175, 216–217) to get an idea of the strength of Frank's motivation to eat less.

FRANK: I want to eat the way I should.

DIETITIAN: Can you give me a number? That helps me understand better where you are with this.

Sometimes people do not assign a number on the first try.

FRANK: I'd say it's a 6 or a 7 for me.

DIETITIAN: You rate it as something of high importance for you. Why didn't you rate it at a 2 or 3?

FRANK: I don't want to mess up my life with more problems. And I need to lose weight.

Change talk

DIETITIAN: Eating better and losing some weight can help you be healthy. Besides getting your glucose more controlled, how else might weight loss help your health?

This reflection connects Frank's desires for better health and weight loss and then continues evoking.

FRANK: I'd probably have more energy, not tired all the time, and feel better about myself.

Change talk

DIETITIAN: I'd like to continue by asking you about how confident you are that you would be successful in losing some weight. On the same scaling system, how confident are you that you would be successful? Zero is not at all confident and 10 is very confident you would be successful.

The rulers gauge readiness for change by exploring both importance and confidence.

FRANK: I'm at a 5 or 6. But it bothers me to say that. I feel like I am someone who can get things done. I've done that in my work and in my relationships with people.

DIETITIAN: Why didn't you rate yourself at a 0 or a 1?

FRANK: This is different than the things I do well. It's more difficult. But last year was one of the first times I was successful with weight loss. And I gained back only 3 of the 12 pounds I lost. With what's happened lately, my weight is down by 19 pounds.

Frank continues to comment on his self-efficacy and feelings he has about this area of his life.

DIETITIAN: You are already seeing success with weight loss. Your worry seems to be based on whether you can eat the way you want to when you are eating alone. What would it take for

The dietitian reflects on Frank's weight loss and continues with another open question based on his confidence.

you to increase your confidence level from a 6 to an 8 or 9?

FRANK: That's a hard question. When we were talking about importance, an idea came to me. I think I'll ask the company if I can do a couple of short trips, just 2 days or so. I think it would be easier to make these changes on a short trip at first. That might help me later on longer trips.

Frank responds with mobilizing change talk, things he could do to change his eating habits.

DIETITIAN: Getting some experience with this makes sense. How would you go about arranging that?

The reflection is followed by an open question exploring steps toward change.

FRANK: I've done a lot for the company over the past 14 years. They appreciate me. I think if I talked to my boss he would OK the idea. I need to do that as soon as possible.

Frank places an urgency on his need to change.

DIETITIAN: That sounds like a great start—to try eating better and swimming on some short trips. Is there anything else you'd like to discuss today?

FRANK: I probably will have other questions after I try this.

DIETITIAN: So, when could we talk again? Could you make an appointment after you complete those two shorter trips? If you have questions before then, just let me know. I will get some booklets for you on choosing foods at fast-food restaurants.

Time to Think

In each of his interviews Frank has had time to think about what he said to his physician and dietitian. Reflective listening and open questions provide time for people to respond, reflect on their experience, and look ahead. Unlike the "yes" or "no" answers to closed questions, open questions ask

Reflective listening and open questions provide time for people to respond, reflect on their experience, and look ahead.

people to think more about their personal details before they answer the question.

The time for patients to think need not make the appointment longer. MI can be used in both brief and longer encounters. Time to think furnishes you with more details about the person's circumstances. Those details include an understanding of the patient's ambivalence, reasons to turn toward or away from change, and the presence of other conditions that may become obstacles standing in the way. In the context of reflective listening, MI provides time and a safe setting for people to conceive plans for change and develop the details of how they will carry out their plans.

The patient-centered momentum of MI gives the lead to the patient, who builds the steps toward better health after providing the reasons for changing the status quo.

Key Points

- Asking permission to discuss sensitive or controversial topics is not just a respectful habit. It honors the patient's autonomy, and in the end, when patients say "Yes" to a conversation, the topic can remain open for discussion at subsequent encounters.

- Reactance is a perceived loss of freedom that causes people to paradoxically cling to unhealthy behaviors while at the same time working on other healthy options. Understanding this paradox and evoking change talk help to avoid the righting reflex, often followed by the patient's justification for unhealthy behaviors.

- Affirmations are especially helpful when people are facing challenging changes.

CHAPTER 8

Physical Activity and Healthy Eating

Managing physical activity and healthy eating are major challenges in the self-care of diabetes. In fact, these areas challenge many people, not just those with diabetes. Considering that people with diabetes face recommendations to exercise 150 minutes weekly (American Diabetes Association, 2014, p. S31) and adhere to a litany of food dicta, it is not hard to understand why some feel overwhelmed and choose to ignore this advice. Even people with a strong interest in change often feel discouragingly far from where they want to be when they try to lose weight or engage in more physical activity.

Avoiding Binary Thinking

Both patients and clinicians can fall prey to the inaccurate and unhelpful view of change as either all or none. This implies a binary perfection standard: success or failure, in the game or out of it, adherence or relapse. This is how New Year's resolutions fail. Successful behavior change tends to be gradual and imperfect: two steps forward and one step back. In the course of a typical day, people may make hundreds of minute-to-minute choices about eating and exercise, and change is about tipping the balance of those choices in a new direction. It is a directional process of approximations toward a desired outcome.

Along the way, there are bound to be fluctuations, like a day of overeating or neglecting other aspects of self-care. Holidays, vacations, and sudden changes in daily routine—an ill family member or car breakdown—disrupt plans. If one neglects to visit the gym this morning, the immediate future offers additional opportunities. Deciding that "I am going to really enjoy a piece of chocolate cake at lunch today" does not negate days of hard work on developing healthier eating habits, nor does it determine future decisions. A key is to avoid discouragement—your own or your patient's—that an exception spells disaster: "Now I've done it! I'm off my diet. I knew I couldn't do it." Nearly everyone working on change makes decisions sometimes that are not consistent with his or her goals. This is normal, and the patient is still free to continue with his or her plan by selecting different options at any future time. Overeating or avoiding planned physical activity is not a question about success or failure. It is an opportunity to discuss decisions that move directionally toward a goal, what the person envisions becoming over time. All steps in the right direction are occasions for affirmation. Each pound lost or several minutes of physical activity are critical steps away from an unhealthy status quo. Changing the status quo for better health is not lost when people do not adhere consistently to a plan each day. It is normal to travel back and forth mentally when people initiate change. In spite of detours from the direction of change, people retain the freedom each day to make choices in the direction of change with each pound lost or each segment of time engaged in exercise.

> *In spite of detours from the direction of change, people retain the freedom each day to make choices in the direction of change with each pound lost or each segment of time engaged in exercise.*

Raising a Sensitive Topic

Complicated obstacles can also put off many people before the conversations begin. Obesity and joint pain hamper physical activity. The attractive nature of food makes it difficult for people who perceive a loss when intake of their favorite foods is threatened. Healthy eating is especially a challenge for people with disordered patterns of eating. There are ways to facilitate engagement in this area. Obesity and dietary indiscretion are sensitive topics. Asking permission and emphasizing respect for the person's autonomy

---

In working with patients who drank excessively I had to change not only my language but also my thinking. It required more than taking the word *relapse* out of my vocabulary. As long as I was thinking in black-and-white terms, I would just be looking for euphemisms for the same thing: a slip, backward sliding, a reversal. Human behavior is much more complex than that, and I finally decided just to describe the behavior itself.

—WRM

can help people ease into discussions—for example: "Would it be all right with you if we discussed weight issues? Many people regard this as a difficult area. I have no intention to create discomfort for you. I strongly believe you are in charge of what you do."

Affirming Steps in the Right Direction

A universal aspect of change is the hard work it involves. Affirming the insights people have about change and their abilities with current and past accomplishments is a basic MI skill. Inquiring about changes made in the past that still are valued provides information for working with a person across extended periods of time. Some practitioners obtain this information during the patient's first visit.

Affirmations fit well when people are facing ambitious challenges. Inquiring about the most difficult or important changes people have made in the past often reveals substantial accomplishments. This information is rich material for affirmations: "The skillful work you did to end years of habitual gambling gave you a great sense of satisfaction and a better life. The experience you have making difficult changes can help you with your diabetes self-care." Affirming accomplishments contributes to strengths-based diabetes care rather than an approach based on deficits: "I can understand your frustration caused by eating high calorie desserts recently. But at your last visit you told me how much more energetic you felt after your A1c level improved. You have capably shown that you have the skills needed to address difficulties with your blood glucose levels."

Physical Activity: A Clinical Example

Zoe is a 32-year-old woman who has had T2D for 8 years. During the past year her A1c has ranged from 8.2% to 9.0%. She is taking three oral medications for diabetes. At her last appointment her nurse practitioner (NP) expressed concerns about her rising A1c level. She suggested Zoe add basal insulin to her other current medications for diabetes and hypertension. Zoe refused insulin and told the NP she would like to start a physical exercise program rather than initiate insulin treatment. After a discussion about the importance of insulin in correcting uncontrolled glycemia, her nurse practitioner referred her to a diabetes educator, a nurse who has interest and expertise in helping people become more physically active. This is Zoe's first appointment to discuss physical activity with the diabetes nurse educator. This excerpt of the interview begins after engaging has taken place and as focusing begins.

DIABETES NURSE EDUCATOR: I know from your NP's referral notes that you have diabetes and are interested in a physical activity program. What do you see as the purpose of this visit today?

The diabetes educator begins with an open question.

ZOE: I'm having trouble with my A1c—it's gone up recently, and it was recommended that I start taking insulin every day. I really don't want to do that. I told my NP I'd like to do something completely different. I'm not ready for insulin. When I was in high school and college, I played tennis four or more times a week. I haven't been all that active since then, except for the time just before and after I was diagnosed with diabetes. I had started playing tennis again to try to get rid of the weight I had gained since college and following a pregnancy. I had diabetes when I was pregnant. And I wanted it to go away. But it didn't. I gave up the tennis when I was told that my diabetes didn't go away after the pregnancy. A new baby and diabetes that didn't go away overwhelmed me. I played tennis for 3 months and then gave it up.

Zoe uses sustain talk about insulin and change talk about her desire to reengage in tennis.

DIABETES NURSE EDUCATOR: Even though you were overwhelmed, you were successful with physical activity—you were able to play tennis for 3 months during a very stressful time in your life. And, as you told me, you are aware of the benefits of exercise in weight reduction.

The diabetes educator's reflections consist of two affirmations. Zoe was able to initiate an activity program during a very challenging set of experiences. Second, she affirms Zoe's insight about the beneficial effects of physical activity on weight loss.

ZOE: I actually enjoyed physical activity. But right now I work a lot and have family responsibilities too—an

Change talk concerning exercise

8-year-old daughter and a husband. It's hard for me to find time for everything.

DIABETES NURSE EDUCATOR: You have many things going on in your life, and all of them are important to you. Could we look more closely at what you would like us to focus on today?

The diabetes educator asks permission to work on the topic(s) they will address in this visit. She is guiding the conversation toward diabetes-related topics. At the same time, she acknowledges there are a number of other areas in Zoe's life competing for her time.

ZOE: Sure. That's what I'm here for.

DIABETES NURSE EDUCATOR: I would like to find out what you feel is the most important area to explore in this visit. I have this "bubble sheet" [Figure 3.1] with several topics on this paper. Each circle contains a topic that you could choose for us to explore today. The topics include monitoring blood glucose levels, developing a more active lifestyle, dealing with diabetes at work, healthy eating, improving conditioning to better participate in sports, or family issues. This last circle says "something else" because you may want to focus on something not mentioned here.

In clearly defining the area(s) that will be explored during the visit, agenda mapping with a bubble chart represents a "metaconversation"—a discussion that helps the practitioner decide what will be talked about during the patient's visit (Miller & Rollnick, 2013, pp. 106–118). The chart hones and speeds up the process of focusing. As described in Chapter 4, the bubble sheet includes a visual list of topics written on "colorful bubbles." These are similar to conversation maps that can be useful in a number of diabetes care areas, including medication options, healthy eating, and physical activity. Among the topics included is one that respects the patient's autonomy, giving him or her the opportunity to select "something else"—an unlisted topic the person feels is more important to discuss.

ZOE: Well, I came here to talk about putting together an activity plan for my diabetes. I can deal with the family responsibilities. Tennis would give me a chance to be with friends and to have some personal time. With all of the things I am doing, I need some personal time.

DIABETES NURSE EDUCATOR: You want time for yourself. And you see tennis as a way to get that needed personal time.

The diabetes educator's reflection focuses on a new area of change talk.

ZOE: That's true. But sometimes I think of how busy I am, and I start feeling bad. I may have gotten myself into more work with what I said at my diabetes appointment. I could have just gone on insulin.

Although Zoe has used change talk in describing her ideas, she still has some ambivalence about what she told her nurse practitioner. Ambivalence about change is normal. It is common for people to experience ambivalence before and even after change has been under way.

DIABETES NURSE EDUCATOR: You feel two ways about this. You could just focus on your diabetes and start insulin, but you also think it's really important to be more physically active and to get more personal time, all of which could help you improve your diabetes self-care.

In the diabetes educator's compound reflection about Zoe's ambivalence, she uses the conjunction but to connect ideas about insulin and her desire to be more physically active. The use of the conjunction but in the reflection places the emphasis on the idea that follows it. The reflection emphasizes the value of the changes Zoe has proposed.

ZOE: I really care more about the idea of getting two things I want and need more than insulin—personal time and playing tennis with friends.

DIABETES NURSE EDUCATOR: So, what would this change in your daily routine look like if you had started doing it a few weeks ago? How would today be different if you had included those things in your life?

These open questions are speculative. They offer Zoe an opportunity to think about possible benefits she could experience if she initiated this change.

ZOE: I could be more efficient than I am now. I would play tennis in the morning for 45 minutes or so 4 days each week. I work four 10-hour days now. But I could easily move to five 8-hour days. With our daughter's school schedule, I'd actually be present in the late afternoons more than I am now.

Zoe begins to structure a plan.

DIABETES NURSE EDUCATOR: You have done some thinking about this. You know what you need to do to be successful with this.

ZOE: I need to do something different than eating more and more. I want to find other ways to take care of myself, or I will just keep gaining weight and taking more medicine for my diabetes. I'd like to get rid of some of the weight I've gained.

DIABETES NURSE EDUCATOR: You clearly want to make this change. How would it feel to start this in the next 2 weeks?

This reflection and open question move the conversation toward activation and taking steps.

ZOE: It will take me a month or so to change my work schedule. But I could start tennis now. I think twice a week would allow me to start at a slower pace.

DIABETES NURSE EDUCATOR: Would it be OK if I offered some advice about what you are doing?

Before giving advice, the diabetes educator asks permission. Respect for the patient's autonomy can strengthen engagement in the discussion.

ZOE: Sure.

DIABETES NURSE EDUCATOR: You've done well putting together a plan that will address your need to become active. I would like to just offer some thoughts about diabetes and insulin. Your A1c is high. You are ready to do what it takes from a physical activity perspective. But there's a strong possibility you may still need insulin. Even with your plan for activity and weight loss, your blood glucose levels may not decrease significantly, and the need for insulin may remain. I want to ask you to do something. Could you monitor your blood glucose three times daily, starting now and as you begin playing tennis? You could measure each day when you wake up and then test before and after one meal each day. The best time for after-meal testing is 2 hours after the meal began. You can alternate the meal you test—breakfast one day, lunch the next day, and supper on the third day. This would help both of us to see how your blood glucose levels respond on exercise days and on the days without exercise. This information can help us to see how your diabetes is doing with this plan. What are your thoughts about what I've just said?

Zoe has a healthful plan for physical activity. But she also has uncontrolled T2D. It is daunting to use physical activity as a main way to control diabetes of a younger person with T2D of over 8 years' duration when the person's A1c is 9%. However, both her NP and diabetes educator believe there is value for Zoe to create her own plan to address her uncontrolled diabetes. Plans are often modified when people learn from their experiences. Follow-up is very important for her. The diabetes educator is supporting her autonomy. But she is also pointing out that blood glucose results should be used to evaluate the effectiveness of her plan. A "can-do" attitude facilitates people's efforts to develop change plans. As a progressive disorder, diabetes involves frequent treatment modifications. This is an important feature of practitioners' advice. Self-monitored blood glucose levels also provide an effective way for people to assess the effectiveness of blood glucose control.

ZOE: It's similar to what my nurse practitioner said. She thought it would be hard for me to fix my diabetes with an exercise plan. But it is something I need to try. It can help me lose weight too. I want to see if I can control my diabetes with a big change, rather than by starting another medication. I can see how measuring my blood glucose is helpful. I will work on that too, but I'm not sure about testing that often every day. I will definitely do it like that on the days I am active and test once or twice on other days.

DIABETES NURSE EDUCATOR: I'd like to review our conversation. You've done a lot of planning today. You're going to change your work schedule over the next month so that you can play tennis four mornings each week. Also, you are looking forward to the personal time you will have with your tennis friends. The fact that this plan and eating smaller quantities may help you lose weight is another important value for you. And you will measure blood glucose levels so that we can see in a month or so how your diabetes is responding to this change. Does this sound accurate to you?

The diabetes educator concludes with a reflective summary, which is a review of the conversation and the plan.

ZOE: Yes . . . it does.

DIABETES NURSE EDUCATOR: You are really a determined person. I am looking forward to seeing you again in a month.

This interview deals with a common topic in the care of T2D. True to the progressive nature of diabetes, Zoe's diabetes has become increasingly more uncontrolled over the past year. She eschews insulin, a frequent sentiment among people with T2D. Insulin could rapidly improve her glycemic control. As her diabetes educator indicated at the conclusion of the interview, the path she has chosen will require a strong commitment to regular exercise and less food intake, difficult tasks for many people. Zoe indicated an understanding that the plan may not avoid the need for insulin.

Should Zoe start insulin now? In addition to her refusal of insulin, there is another consideration. There is value in supporting the efforts of a motivated person as she works to change the foundation of her current lifestyle to achieve better diabetes health. Close follow-up is essential. It provides an opportunity to explore adjustments to the plan as needed over time. Most clinical encounters in diabetes perennially involve readjustments in treatments. Zoe is willing to participate actively in follow-up.

Disordered Eating: A Clinical Example

Restrictions related to food are particularly difficult for people with diabetes. In addition to life-sustaining nourishment, mealtimes provide families and friends with time to socialize. Food is an integral part of celebrating holidays, anniversaries, and birthdays. It is also used to help reinforce cultural and religious values. Likewise a major concern of public health organizations worldwide is the overconsumption of simple sugars, starches, and fats that has resulted in vast numbers of overweight and obese people and increases in the incidence of prediabetes and diabetes. The following dialogue addresses weight and disordered eating habits.

Allan, a 43-year-old man, was diagnosed with T2D 3 years earlier. He has a body mass index (BMI) of 36 kg/m² and a strong family history of T2D and obesity. He has successfully lost 4–9% of his weight numerous times. But on each occasion, he regained more weight than he had lost. He is on several medications that he takes appropriately. His A1c is 7.6%. This conversation took place at his last appointment with his physician. After a warm greeting, the process of focusing begins.

PHYSICIAN: You've done good work since your last appointment. Your A1c improved. It dropped from 8.4% to 7.6%.

The physician affirms the improvement in Allan's A1c level.

ALLAN: It's probably because I went on a low-carb diet. But I couldn't lose any weight. There's a lot of fatty food in the diet, and I found myself snacking a lot more.

We will see that Allan and the physician are involved in focusing.

PHYSICIAN: Your weight and diet are frustrating for you. Your concerns are on target, high-fat foods at mealtime and for snacks cause weight gain.

The reflection is strengthened by adding emotion, frustration. The physician provides an affirmation about Allan's insight. What Allan said about his eating moves the conversation toward focusing.

ALLAN: As I told you in the past, I started eating a lot as a kid and have struggled with it ever since. I've also been under more stress. My wife's job was cut to half-time. And at my job I'm struggling with a difficult coworker who's not doing a good job on work I need for a big project.

Eating has been a long-standing issue for Allan.

PHYSICIAN: You have a lot of stress now. I recall you telling me in the past that your weight is influenced by stress. Can you help me understand how food helps you when you're stressed?

The physician ends the complex reflection and makes a statement about past history and then uses an open question to evoke a better understanding of Allan's eating habits.

ALLAN: I'm not real sure about that either. I've been successful at times with weight loss. Sometimes I start gaining weight again because I just like to snack a lot. I really enjoy eating. But most of the time the weight gain has occurred when I'm stressed—like the time my daughter's asthma became severe. She had to be hospitalized. She did well. But we ended up with a lot of expenses that troubled us for about 3 years.

He can lose weight in some situations, but when stress occurs any desire he has to control eating fades.

PHYSICIAN: Stress is a part of life that is difficult for you. That's when you use food to soothe stress.

The conversation expands the focus to include disordered eating.

ALLAN: My childhood was pretty difficult, very stressful. My parents fought all the time. After bad arguments my mother would often make sweets—cakes, cookies, and stuff like that to make up for everything that was going on at home. I'd eat a lot of that stuff. Maybe that's when I got into eating to feel better. Their arguments were painful.

Food ameliorates stress for him.

PHYSICIAN: Would it be OK with you if I shared with you a thought about your eating?

The physician asks permission to discuss a sensitive topic.

ALLAN: Sure. I know I'm overweight. I also hate getting sweaty. So, please don't ask me about using exercise to deal with my weight.

Allan qualifies the consent he is giving to the physician.

PHYSICIAN: I assure you, I won't talk about exercise. The thought I have is about eating associated with weight gain, stress, and diabetes. Using food to control stress is not like the usual social or nutritional aspects of eating. It uses food in a way that can injure your health. But there is something more important than my thoughts about this. I'm interested in what you think about this idea. Your viewpoint is more important than mine.

As the interview continues, Allan states that he has never spoken with anyone about the heavy eating that accompanies his stress. He sees it as a problem and has tried everything he could think of to avoid it. The physician responds with a question.

PHYSICIAN: You want to find a solution to this. What would your life be like if you could better manage this area?

Allan did not indicate he was ready to do something about his eating. The physician uses his reflection "to guess" about his intentions. Guesses elicit more discussion.

ALLAN: That's a hard question. I've always had a real attraction to eating, and I'm unable to resist food when I'm stressed. If I were able to deal with this successfully, I'd probably feel a lot better about myself.

PHYSICIAN: Do you have any ideas about things that could help you change this part of your life?

Allan has used change talk throughout the interview. The interviewer begins to explore Allan's readiness to begin the process of planning.

ALLAN: I don't know. I've never had any success with this even though I really would like to be successful.

PHYSICIAN: You seem uncertain about what you could do. Would it be helpful if I offered you some ideas and advice?

This is an example of elicit–provide–elicit (E-P-E). After asking permission to offer input the interviewer provides information (ideas) and/or advice. Information and advice differ in that the former involves knowledge, data, or research, whereas the latter involves the practitioner's opinions (e.g., what might work better or worse in these circumstances).

ALLAN: I'd like to hear what you have to say.

PHYSICIAN: I am concerned that your eating is not just related to enjoying food. You feel compelled to eat when you're under stress, and that falls into the category of disordered eating. Disordered eating often does not go away, even when people would like it to. You certainly have worked hard on it, but you're not satisfied with how you've been dealing with this issue. One way you could address this would be with a psychologist. She or he could help you explore this area and work on it productively. A second approach would be to speak with

E-P-E is used here with respect for autonomy. The physician offers options and includes as the last choice not addressing disordered eating at all. Honoring autonomy offers people time to think about options. When people feel their autonomy is being threatened by a list of choices that do not work for them, there is a risk they may feel misunderstood and resentful of the

a dietitian who is a diabetes educator. They know a lot about healthy eating. But this would not address your history of food use as a way to soothe stress. And, of course, you always have the option of not doing anything about it. What are your thoughts about these options?

interviewer's intrusion and focus on those sentiments instead of considering change.

E-P-E always ends with an invitation to the client to share his or her opinions about the options.

ALLAN: I'm not sure what to say. You're saying that the way I eat when I'm stressed is a mental problem. I've never thought of it that way in the past. And I've never thought I'd have to see a psychologist for help with my eating. I've always thought that I could handle things pretty well in my life.

PHYSICIAN: You're a capable person; you work hard to take care of your diabetes. What I heard you say earlier is that you don't feel like you have a way to address stress and eating. Listening to you suggests to me you may want to do something about this area of your life. You'd like to find a way to do something about the effect of stress on your weight.

The physician uses an affirmation—"You are a capable person"—and follows up with a reflection about Allan's difficulties in addressing stress and his eating habits. It respectfully places the onus of developing a solution on Allan.

ALLAN: I'd like to think you're right. But I never thought of this area of my life as a mental problem. But maybe that's why I haven't solved this problem. I will think about your suggestion. Could I get back with you about this?

The first step in initiating change is to think about it. This change talk statement is an example of commitment language.

PHYSICIAN: That sounds like a good idea. Thinking about this challenging area of your life is important. How do you want to follow up on this?

The physician offers an open question at the end of the statement. As a commitment to change is considered, open questions provide people with a way to elaborate on ideas related to their commitment. This open question deals with remaining engaged and focused on what to do about this important obstacle to weight loss.

ALLAN: Your appointment schedule is usually booked out too far. I could email you in the next week. If I decide to see a psychologist, I'll need names.

Allan offers an easier choice than attempting to get another appointment. This gives him room for ambivalence and also time to think about seeking treatment for his disordered eating habits.

PHYSICIAN: That sounds good. I know a person that I think you'd enjoy working with. One more thing: because of the logjam with appointments, please get a date to check in with me in 3 months.

Rather than pushing Allan to make a commitment in a sensitive area, the physician opts to focus on the follow-up interval for his next appointment. The topic remains open if Allan forgoes emailing him.

Allan is not prepared to initiate a plan now, but he is willing to consider it. This is the first step in commitment: considering change, followed by how the plan could be accomplished. Allan also took a big step—he committed himself to email his thoughts about seeing a therapist.

Disordered overeating is a common obstacle in diabetes. Teenagers, especially girls, with T1D often omit insulin to cover snacks and meals to

Disordered overeating is a common obstacle in diabetes.

avoid weight gain. Also disordered overeating is often encountered in T2D. Disordered eating can present as an insurmountable problem, a difficult health condition that many are not trained to treat. Disordered eating falls under the purview of mental health practitioners because these conditions are more likely to be successfully treated by psychologists and other mental health professionals than by diabetes practitioners.

Both of the interviewers in this chapter used reflective listening, a skill that uses reflections more than questions. When people hear reflections of what they have just said, it provides an opportunity for them to think about what they just said. The skillful use of reflections also provides a more detailed understanding of the client's circumstances. This approach is critically important in the evoking process—evoking the person's own reasons and plans for initiating change.

Two or three reflections followed by an open-ended question often create a pleasant rhythm for MI interviews. It is a rhythm that is free of discord. It eliminates the need for the righting reflex and other persuasive attempts to "install change." It is a rhythm conducive to considering change.

Key Points

- Behavior change is not a binary process leading to failure or success. It is a directional approximation toward a desired outcome.

- Affirmations of people's past or current achievements or insights are especially helpful when people are facing difficult changes.

- Diabetes health care is a team sport. When patients have a history of disordered patterns of eating, they are unlikely to be successfully treated by diabetes professionals. Mental health professionals can fill a huge void in diabetes care by helping people work on obstacles—disordered eating and other mental health conditions—that stand in the way of better diabetes outcomes.

- Reflective listening is a foundational skill for MI. It offers an opportunity to learn more about the details of people's lives. It is also helpful for evoking the patient's ideas and solutions for improving self-care.

CHAPTER 9

Medication Use

Think of the large amount of time spent discussing medications in diabetes health care. People facing the chronic use of medications raise concerns about drugs. Many of them discuss medications in terms of what is desired or not desired. Even though the number of effective drugs for diabetes is greater now than ever before, many people remain skeptical about using them.

Some patients take a minimalist approach:

"I'd rather take care of diabetes naturally by watching what I eat and being more active. I would use medications only if I had complications."

"I don't think cholesterol-lowering drugs are very safe. I've heard about the liver and muscle problems they can cause. I'd rather change my diet instead."

"I've read that aspirin can be dangerous. It causes me to bruise easily, and I'd rather not take it."

Others take a selective approach:

"If I have to be on a second medicine, I'd rather take the one you inject—the one that helps people lose weight."

"I'm willing to take some of these medicines you're talking about, but if you're planning to put me on insulin, I can't do it. I don't want to get to that point with my diabetes."

Among practitioners, a large emphasis is placed on prescribing particular medications and providing information and counseling about their use. Clinical practice guidelines (American Diabetes Association, 2014; American Association of Endocrinologists, 2013) provide algorithms for recommending medications and research that further refines information about diabetes treatments (Brown & Bussell, 2011). These reports are aimed directly at diabetes practitioners. Companies laud their patented drugs in advertisements that appear in countless diabetes journals and newsletters. And, importantly, the compassionate feelings of practitioners centered on helping people avoid preventable suffering motivate frequent conversations about medications with patients. Yet, all the time spent on discussing this topic does not diminish the somber finding that people with diabetes end up skipping many doses of their medications (Cramer, 2004).

MI and Medication Adherence

Research also demonstrates that MI is an effective way to help people deal with their use of medications, offering practitioners a valuable way to address this important area of diabetes care. MI has been helpful in studies on medication adherence in depression (Kaplan, Keeley, Engel, Emsermann, & Brody, 2013; Lewis-Fernández et al., 2013), hypertension (Ogedegbe et al., 2008), thought disorders (Hamrin & McGuinness, 2013), and AIDs (Hill & Kavookjian, 2012). MI has a generic quality that enables its use to fit into many different settings.

Two landmark diabetes studies demonstrated the value of conscientiously using two basic diabetes medications: insulin and metformin. There were powerful benefits for people with diabetes using these medications. In the Diabetes Control and Complications Trial (DCCT) the intensive use of insulin in T1D was tested. The United Kingdom Prospective Diabetes Study (UKPDS) tested metformin and numerous other oral medications as well as insulin in T2D patients. Importantly, these studies showed the negative outcomes often resulting from diabetes could be sizably improved by the efficacious use of insulin in T1D and metformin in T2D.

The DCCT showed impressive outcomes in T1D treatment when insulin was used intensively to lower A1c levels. In the primary prevention group (using the intensive insulin treatment regimen), the risk of diabetic retinopathy was reduced by 76%. In the secondary prevention group the risk of retinopathy progressing to proliferative retinopathy (the eye disorder that causes blindness in diabetes) was reduced by 54%. In both the primary and secondary prevention cohorts, treatment with intensive insulin therapy lowered the development of diabetic kidney disease by 39% and the occurrence of clinical neuropathy by 60% (Diabetes Control and Complications Trial Research Group, 1993). In the second study, the UKPDS, those allocated to the treatment group that used metformin for blood glucose control in A1c experienced a 42% risk reduction for diabetes-related death and a 36% reduction in the risk for all-cause mortality (UKPDS Study Group, 1998).

Two large categories of medications are used to treat people with diabetes. The first group of diabetes drugs treats the metabolic imbalances created by hyperglycemia. Metformin and insulin are common drugs in this group. Second are the drugs that address prevention or amelioration of secondary complications. Examples include statins, used to prevent myocardial infarctions and stroke, and angiotensin-converting enzyme inhibitors (ACE inhibitors) or angiotensin receptor blockers (ARBs), drugs used to treat hypertension or congestive heart failure. They are also used to attempt to prevent diabetic kidney disease.

The Spirit of MI

Imagine a person with T2D named Sharon, who, after reading about statins, believes that the potential side effects of them might outweigh the benefits of delaying or avoiding cardiovascular complications, a stroke, or myocardial infarction from diabetes-related causes. And think of the contrasts between using the righting reflex in lieu of the spirit of MI (see Chapter 2) in a conversation about this topic with Sharon. The motivation of a practitioner using the righting reflex might look like this: "It's really important for Sharon to understand the significance of statin use for helping her live a longer and more comfortable life with diabetes."

The practitioner working within the spirit of MI, on the other hand, is curious about how someone would elect the high risks of serious cardiovascular events rather than the risks of drug complications that are extraordinarily rare. Using MI, the interviewer is thinking, "This person surely has reasons supporting her willingness to risk the dreaded, common occurrences of heart attack or stroke. Listening and understanding her point of view might be challenging, but it will also be interesting." The practitioner's curiosity is understandable, since the risk of myocardial infarction in people with diabetes is three to four times greater than in people without diabetes.

Along with his or her curiosity, the practitioner using MI also has an underlying sense of acceptance of the patient and respect for his or her autonomy. But rather than convincing Sharon that statins are a good treatment, he or she wants to collaboratively explore her thoughts about this issue. The practitioner listens closely in order to better treat the disease, realizing that in order to provide treatment he must first understand her. Understanding her motivations for avoiding statins is facilitated by using reflective listening. The practitioner wants to know even more: Does this person have a strong

> *Along with his or her curiosity, the practitioner using MI also has an underlying sense of acceptance of the patient and respect for his or her autonomy.*

opinion of avoiding statins, or is there some ambivalence about that position? The answer will be revealed by the presence or absence of change talk in Sharon's statements. If change talk is absent, it will be difficult to evoke it with language that does not also embody compassion, empathy, and acceptance on his part.

Creating Discrepancy

MI, an ideal fit for resolving a patient's ambivalence, can also be used to *create* ambivalence. This is especially useful when working with people who are adhering to the status quo. In MI, this is referred to as creating a discrepancy. Discrepancy is essentially a gap between the person's values and where he or she is today in a specific area of his or her life.

> MI, *an ideal fit for resolving a patient's ambivalence, can also be used to create ambivalence.*

For example, you are working with someone in late-middle age who is struggling with glycemic control. He also speaks longingly of retiring in 10 years. If the conversation is focused on glycemic issues, it would be helpful to use what he had previously said in framing an open-ended question: "I can understand your interest in retiring. You speak of it so positively. You are really looking forward to it. But I'm wondering how your A1c of 9.8% fits into that plan?" This is stated respectfully, without sarcasm.

The question asks him to think about where he is and where he wants to be in the future. It often results in the rapid assembly of the person's internal "ambivalence committee." That committee has strong voices that argue with one another. In this case it says, "I'm dreaming up great plans for retirement, but the challenges of taking care of my diabetes could actually mess up my future." The patient picks up on what he is hearing himself think and says, "I need to do something about my blood glucose levels." When you hear change talk, even if it is quite weak, the conversation can begin to explore the resolution of ambivalence. A response to the previous statement could be: "I know what you mean. It would be difficult not being able to participate fully in your important plans. What I'm hearing is that part of you is struggling with blood glucose control, but there is also another part of you that really wants to do something about it." An additional example of creating discrepancy appears in the second interview with Sharon, below.

Amid their busy schedules providing health care to people with diabetes, practitioners often make statements that can generate understandable concerns. These statements signal a need for more time to discuss the concerns raised by the patients' hesitancy to use medications. And even though medications can ameliorate the metabolic dysfunctions of diabetes and help people delay or avoid complications, patients often focus more on potential side effects, and as a result do not take them. Other barriers—the significant expenses and/or the large number of recommended medications—make this area even more challenging.

This chapter examines contrasting interview styles through a dialogue with Sharon, a 56-year-old woman who has had T2D for 3 months. She is reluctant to start using a statin medication for her elevated LDL cholesterol level. The first interview is not MI-based, while the second one is. The two interviewers are physician assistants who work in diabetes care.

Non-MI Interview Addressing Cardiovascular Risk

PHYSICIAN ASSISTANT: How have you been doing, Sharon?

SHARON: I finished increasing my metformin dose a few weeks ago, and my blood glucose levels have been close to what you told me they should be. And I'm not having stomachaches from the medicine anymore.

Sharon focuses on her success with blood glucose management, and is taking her metformin as prescribed.

PHYSICIAN ASSISTANT: That sounds good. We downloaded your blood glucose meter, and the values are right where they should be. I'm also glad to see your weight has not increased. It's down a little bit—3 pounds. How many times each week are you involved in physical activity?

The physician assistant acknowledges her success with blood glucose management and mentions that she has not gained weight and then asks a closed question.

SHARON: Two or 3 days a week for about a half an hour. I'm walking sometimes in the morning and sometimes in the evening.

Sharon is walking 90 minutes weekly, less than the recommended 150 minutes weekly.

PHYSICIAN ASSISTANT: Two additional days of physical activity would provide a better impact on your blood glucose levels. Also early-in-the-day physical activity influences your blood glucose more than late-in-the-day exercise.

Advice about the need for additional time walking each week and the benefits of walking in the morning. Advice is provided without seeking permission.

SHARON: I go to work early in the morning. I can't afford to be late.

Sharon argues for maintaining physical activity in the evening.

PHYSICIAN ASSISTANT: I would like to pick up where we left off in the appointment 2 months ago. We discussed your need to take a statin, the medicine that lowers your LDL cholesterol levels, the bad cholesterol that causes heart attacks. You had concerns about doing that, so I asked you to think about it. Your level of LDL is quite high, you know. Have you decided to use this medication?

The physician assistant continues to focus on questions he has. The physician assistant provides a good reason for Sharon to be on a statin.

SHARON: I haven't changed my mind. I still have concerns about what I have read about those drugs. They can cause muscle damage, and some people die from that.

Notwithstanding her elevated LDL level, Sharon puts aside the physician assistant's persuasion and says she will not take a statin.

PHYSICIAN ASSISTANT: Having a heart attack can be fatal, too. And that occurs far more frequently in people with diabetes than death from statins. Statins very rarely cause death!

The physician assistant uses fear, hoping it will help convince Sharon to be on a statin.

SHARON: They can also cause liver damage.

Sharon leaves aside the benefits of statins and comments on other problems associated with them. When arguments occur in health care encounters, both health care providers and patients often feel bad about the encounter.

PHYSICIAN ASSISTANT: The elevation of liver enzymes is rare. We know your liver function tests are normal now, and I don't think you have much to worry about with this. Most of the side effects of statins do not cause death or disability. But heart attacks and strokes often cause that.

Disagreement and persuasion continues.

SHARON: I don't see myself taking something like that. I would rather work on my diet and try being more physically active.

Sharon uses change talk about another approach.

PHYSICIAN ASSISTANT: Heart attacks kill more people than any other disease. People with diabetes have a risk of heart attack two to three or four times that of people without diabetes. Wouldn't you feel better if you were taking something that could lower that risk?

Instilling fear does not usually facilitate change. It can encourage avoidance or a desire to escape.

SHARON: Not now. As I just told you, I have a plan.

Sharon reiterates her position on statin use.

PHYSICIAN ASSISTANT: It would be good for you to do the things you are suggesting, but they don't provide the same cardiovascular protection that statins do. You could make your plan a lot more reliable by adding a statin.

SHARON: So? I have to live my own life. I do things differently. I'll tell you one thing: I can take care of my diabetes. You said so yourself when we got started today in this discussion.

Listen! I'm not going to do this!

PHYSICIAN ASSISTANT: But it's important for people with diabetes to get the best treatment. I would not be doing my job if I did not emphasize how important this area of diabetes care really is. I'd like you to think more about this decision. At your next appointment 3 months from now we can continue this conversation. I'm going to give you some reading material that may change your mind.

This truism about the importance of "best treatment" is another effort to persuade Sharon.

SHARON: Look, I'm not going to take a medicine to lower my cholesterol. I'm happy, however, to discuss other areas of my diabetes. I don't feel like moving on this topic.

I'm not sure I need any reading material. I have already read about those medicines.

The more Sharon is pushed, the more forcefully she pushes back.

PHYSICIAN ASSISTANT: That's unfortunate. I will indicate in your chart the decision you are making not to use a medication for your elevated "bad [LDL] cholesterol" level. I will probably bring this up again. It's an important part of good health care, and I want you to have the best outcomes possible with your diabetes.

In this conversation Sharon responded by arguing in favor of an unhealthy option, not taking a statin. MI focuses on evoking change talk toward health rather than perpetuating sustain talk for continuing a less healthy choice.

MI Interview Addressing Cardiovascular Risk

PHYSICIAN ASSISTANT: It's good to see you again, Sharon. How have you been doing since your last appointment?

The physician assistant greets her and begins with an open question.

SHARON: I finished increasing my metformin dose a few weeks ago, and my blood glucose levels have been close to what you told me they should be. And I'm not having stomachaches from the medicine anymore.

PHYSICIAN ASSISTANT: That's really good to hear. You're checking your blood glucoses twice daily, and I see the progress you've made with your glucose values when you reached the target dose of metformin. You're working hard with the medication, and it also sounds like you're feeling more confident about the care for your diabetes.

Unlike the prior interview, he follows up reflectively and adds an affirmation: "You're working hard with the medication, and it also sounds like you're feeling more confident . . . . "

SHARON: I'm a lot more confident that things will work out well for me. I am glad my blood glucose levels have dropped. My eating habits have changed since I visited the dietitian.

PHYSICIAN ASSISTANT: It sounds as though you are working a lot on your diabetes. How can I help you today?

The physician assistant uses an open question to facilitate focusing.

SHARON: The diabetes educator spoke with me about exercise, and I'm walking two or three times a week. I'm enjoying the walks—they feel good.

PHYSICIAN ASSISTANT: You're working to eat better and are controlling your blood glucose levels well. And you've started walking. You have a lot of insight on healthy ways to control diabetes.

An affirmation follows the reflections.

SHARON: I do feel better.

PHYSICIAN ASSISTANT: Would it be all right if I brought up a topic we discussed at your last appointment—lowering your LDL cholesterol and your risks of heart attacks and strokes?

The physician assistant asks permission before inquiring about a sensitive topic.

SHARON: I'm willing to discuss it, but I have strong feelings about not taking that medicine.

PHYSICIAN ASSISTANT: I understand what you're saying. But this conversation is not taking place to make you do something. I'm unable to do that. It is your diabetes, and only you can make the decisions about how you're going to take care of it.

The physician assistant shows respect for Sharon's autonomy.

SHARON: I like that idea.

PHYSICIAN ASSISTANT: We talked last time about how people with diabetes have significantly elevated risks for heart attacks and strokes . . . and you had reservations about taking statins to lower the risks. What you told me at the last appointment and what I'm hearing now tells me you are not at all interested in statins. The risks of these complications don't concern you. You feel you should never use statins.

The physician assistant comes alongside with a reflection that mirrors Sharon's own opinion that statins are too dangerous for her to use. Coming alongside is a last-ditch approach for evoking change talk (Miller & Rollnick, 2013, p. 199).

SHARON: That's not exactly what I said. I know these risks are real. My father had a heart attack and almost died. For the rest of his life he had heart failure. And one of my grandmothers had a bad stroke—she ended up in a nursing home. I don't want my life to end like theirs did. But I live in much more healthy fashion than my father and grandmother. Both of them smoked. But I feel good now. I definitely don't want to get sick from the side effects of a drug.

Sharon begins to qualify where she is. Before the conclusion of what she says here, she uses change talk, expressing what she wants in her life: "I don't want my life to end like theirs did."

PHYSICIAN ASSISTANT: You want to use caution. That's understandable. Dealing with your diabetes is hard work, and you don't want to end up with another chronic condition caused by a drug.

The reflective listening continues.

SHARON: Exactly.

PHYSICIAN ASSISTANT: You have a family history of heart attack and stroke. You've recently developed type 2 diabetes, and you're 56 years old. As you think about your life, what do you want it to look like when you are retired 10 or so years from now? What do you want to be doing then?

SHARON: I want to be healthy and have my diabetes controlled well. I want to be able to travel with my husband and visit our grandchildren and their parents, our kids. I want to be able to help our son and daughters with their kids when they need a break. We have one son and two daughters. Seeing them involves a day or two of travel from here. And the good news is we may be able to retire in 8 years.

PHYSICIAN ASSISTANT: You and your husband are already making plans, lovely plans for a promising future.

SHARON: And we are taking a lot more short vacations now to visit them. Getting diabetes has me a bit worried, but I've always been able to manage tough times in my life.

PHYSICIAN ASSISTANT: Several times today you've brought up the importance of doing a good job with your diabetes. That attitude is strong. From what you told me in the last visit, you have a long history of managing things that most people find difficult.

In lieu of questions or advice, the physician assistant continues with reflective listening. Sharon responds with lots of details about her life and her aspirations.

SHARON: I get that from my parents.

PHYSICIAN ASSISTANT: Family figures importantly in your life. Your parents and your offspring have given you a lot to live for. As you look 8 to 10 years down the road, how do you fit the risk of a heart attack or stroke into the plans you have made?

The physician assistant chooses to ask an important question, one that might elicit ambivalent statements. This question highlights Sharon's values and a potential discrepancy— becoming too ill or dying before enjoying retirement.

SHARON: I want to be able to be healthy as long as possible. But I'm worried about the side effects of the drug I would have to take. So I don't like the idea of those medicines. But I also feel like I need a life after I retire. And I want to do what I can to make that happen.

Sharon responds with change talk: "I also feel like I need a life after I retire." And she follows with more change talk: "And I want to do what I can to make that happen." These statements express a reason ("need a life after I retire") and a desire ("I want to do what I can to make that happen") to change. They are her first change talk statements.

PHYSICIAN ASSISTANT: I hear you saying two things. You want to avoid a helpful medication that potentially has side effects. And another part of you is saying you're curious about statins because they might be helpful to you.

The physician assistant hears the ambivalence and continues with reflections that focus on it.

SHARON: I guess so. I really don't want to be on a statin. But I need to be alive in order to enjoy my family. I'm feeling stuck with this decision making. I feel like I have to make myself be curious about something I am struggling with.

PHYSICIAN ASSISTANT: You need to do what works best for you. I can't force this on you. Would it be helpful for me to give you an idea of how likely medication problems are compared to the likelihood of a heart attack?

The physician assistant clearly indicates that Sharon is the one who will make this decision. But he also asks her permission to provide information that may be helpful to her.

SHARON: Yes, I have very mixed feelings about the drug but no mixed feelings about the value of my family.

Sharon reveals her ambivalence with a brief statement that expresses uncertainty about the statin and strong positive statements about her family.

PHYSICIAN ASSISTANT: The risk of a heart attack for a 56-year-old woman with diabetes and your cholesterol and BP levels and no smoking is 27% [Risk Score Profiles, 2013]. With realistic outcomes, and taking a statin to lower your LDL level, the risk would be 11% [Risk Score Profiles, 2013]. The annual risk of serious muscle side effects, the kind that can lead to death, occurs in less than 5 people out of 100,000. Milder, nonlethal forms of muscle pain occur in about 10–15% of people, many of whom

Elicit–provide–elicit (E-P-E) is used to provide this information. After receiving permission, the physician assistant offers the information and ends with an open question, "What are your thoughts about this information?"

recover spontaneously. Some of them discontinue the drug. The liver side effects from a statin are rare and are hardly ever associated with damage to the liver [Maji, Shaika, Solanki, & Gaurav, 2013]. Blood tests you have recently had show no evidence of liver problems. And they will be very unlikely. What are your thoughts about this information?

SHARON: The risk of heart attack is a lot higher than I expected, and the drug problems are much less frequent than I thought they would be. It's like good news/bad news.

PHYSICIAN ASSISTANT: The frequency of heart disease creates the emphasis on reducing its risk in diabetes. Those events are much more common in people with diabetes than the rest of the population. But it's your decision to do what you want to about this set of circumstances.

When autonomy is respected, people have no need to argue. Instead, they have time to think about the decision.

SHARON: I need to make a decision about this. I want to be in the game as long as possible. Let me discuss this with my husband and think about it a bit more. Could I come back later this month?

Sharon has journeyed away from status quo to ambivalence. She realizes the importance of considering this area. She is putting together an early step in commitment, thinking about what change would look like.

PHYSICIAN ASSISTANT: Sure. Write down any questions that come up. It's important to get your questions answered.

SHARON: I will make an appointment. I appreciate speaking with you about this, and I like having some time to think about what to do. I still have fears about side effects. But I don't favor dying early either. I want to be here.

Who Told Sharon What to Do?

What differences do you perceive in these two interviews? A couple of hints for answering this question relate to persuasion and the contrasts in agenda setting in the interviews. The skills (OARS) and the spirit of MI offer a way to put aside the righting reflex, an attempt to convince through persuasion or emphatic arguments that change is essential. The differences in agenda setting are significant. The agenda in the first interview was set by the interviewer only. He aimed "to get Sharon on a statin." But he neglected a salient fact: There is only one person that you can "get to change"—namely, yourself. And people initiate change only when they are ready, willing, and able to do so. If that readiness is not present, trying to force people to do something does not work.

There are many opportunities in diabetes care to help people prevent complications and enhance their self-care. Sometimes, as in the first interview, the righting reflex is used and people are just persuasively told what to do. But this works well for only a minority of people, those who arrive for their appointments ready to initiate change before the discussion begins.

Many people, however, are not ready to initiate change. They do not respond well to arguments, pleas, or recommendations to make changes in their self-care. Because of these barriers, simply telling them what to do does not work. Some are comfortable with their status quo. Others have significant ambivalence. Others may be facing difficult barriers—depression, chemical dependency disorders, or eating disorders. Often they do not complain when the righting reflex is used. They simply leave appointments and return to the next visit in the same compromised self-care circumstances they were in at their previous appointment. Even when the righting reflex is used with conviction, change is deferred. Working with people in this fashion may result in long periods of compromised self-care. Their follow-up appointments are a litany of status quo or ambivalent statements of how difficult or distasteful change is. Even worse, some of these people disengage from health care services altogether.

MI is a more tactful person-centered approach. In place of the righting reflex, MI evokes discussions and guides the conversations away from interpersonal controversy, arguments, and persuasion. The appointment becomes "an active collaboration between experts" (Miller & Rollnick, 2013, p. 29) who are discussing change, an expert in diabetes and the other an expert in him- or herself.

In conversations using MI, the personal experts do not develop their own plans on a whim or wish or persuasion. Instead, they have an opportunity to think and explore change in a compassionate environment where partnership and autonomy are respected. The spirit and skills of MI create an opportunity for people like Sharon. In the second interview above, she wound up telling herself what she would do and yet did not experience a moment during the interview when she felt the need to respond reactively to being told what to do.

Key Points

- Attempting to "install change" with the righting reflex often fails. The spirit of MI, OARS, and curiosity helps with understanding why a person argues for an unhealthy status quo.
- Understanding the patient's position makes it easier to evoke change talk.
- Creating a discrepancy actually creates ambivalence when working with people adherent to the status quo. The discrepancy is a gap between where they are now and what they would value in the future.

CHAPTER 10

Insulin Use in Type 2 Diabetes

People newly diagnosed with T2D are often relieved when they learn that the only medications they need for their diabetes can be taken orally. Most people with T2D would like to avoid insulin, and if it is needed later on they may feel as though lapses in their self-care are to blame: "I just didn't try hard enough. Before starting insulin, I need a chance to do better." In essence, this is what Zoe said in Chapter 8. Similar expressions of self-blame are commonly heard in busy diabetes practices.

Although healthy behaviors can facilitate blood glucose control, over time they may not prevent the need for insulin. The progressive nature of diabetes involves regular modifications of treatments in order to avoid diabetic complications.

Lifestyle changes and medications are important parts of diabetes self-care. Research has shown that a series of healthy behaviors related to lifestyle issues and medication use can actually prevent or palliate diabetic complications (Diabetes Control and Complications Trial Research Group, 1993; UKPDS Study Group, 1998). Although lifestyle changes alone can prevent the development of diabetes (Diabetes Prevention Program Research Group, 2002), a cogent argument maintains that intensifying lifestyle modifications alone does not effectively treat uncontrolled diabetes (Schellenberg, Dryden, Vandermeer, Ha, & Korownyk, 2013). Treatment with insulin is often needed to manage T2D in the long run.

There are numerous oral and injectable medications other than insulin that improve glycemic control in T2D, but none of them possesses the efficacy of insulin, a drug with almost a century of history helping people better control their diabetes. Insulin fills the gap, as endogenous insulin production is exhausted over time by the metabolic problems of diabetes. The likelihood of needing it comes sooner for people who are diagnosed later in the course of having T2D. Their insulin levels wane more rapidly after diagnosis than in people diagnosed earlier in the course of the disease.

Although people sometimes lament the start of insulin treatment, even those initially opposed to using it often feel better after they begin to do so. Once people with T2D start taking insulin they seldom look back or talk about discontinuing it. As their blood glucose levels improve their energy levels increase. The satisfaction of being better able to better control glucose levels is also more satisfying and provides patients with a sense of accomplishment. These positive impacts are common with a treatment that paradoxically seems threatening or undesirable.

Reflective listening and evoking can be effective skills to use when talking to a patient about using insulin.

Reflective Listening

Reflective listening (first described in Chapter 5) begins with concentrating attentively on what is being said, listening for helpful information about the patient's motivations and readiness for change. Reflective listening frees you from trying to come up with your next question or clever refutation. Instead, you work in the fashion of a translator, concentrating on understanding what the patient means. Your thoughts might look like this: "He just said this. I think he means much more than what he actually said. So, I am going to tell him what I think I heard and also what I think this means to him." This type of thinking formulates a complex reflection.

Miller and Rollnick have offered a visual metaphor for understanding how reflections work. They described the creation of reflections as something similar to an iceberg (Miller & Rollnick, 2013, p. 58). Simple reflections—merely repeating what the patient has already said—are like the tip of the iceberg, the part above the water, while complex reflections make a guess about what is still hidden under the water. Consider this example: Patient: "I don't like the idea of taking insulin. I just need to work harder to improve my A1c."

> Simple Reflection: "You don't want to take insulin, and you're willing to work hard on better control of your diabetes."

This type of reflection merely repeats what the patient has already said. It might be good enough, but a complex reflection is more likely to move the discussion forward.

A complex reflection is more likely to move the discussion forward.

> Complex reflection: "You want to get your A1c level down to stay healthy; that's really important to you. Starting insulin seems like a big step, and you're wondering if you can put it off a while by trying harder."

This complex reflection opens up the discussion in several ways. It starts by emphasizing the positive—the patient's desire to control his or her A1c level and be healthy. It also reframes the patient's negative statement about insulin into more a matter of wondering. Chances are the patient does have some doubt about whether "trying harder" would be enough. Note that a reflection does not disagree with what the patient has said.

It is often easier to facilitate change by reflecting instead of asking questions. Imagine the patient's response in this situation if you had asked, "Why don't you want to start insulin?" or "Do you really think you can get your A1c down by trying harder?" Reflective listening engages the patient in the problem-solving process. It prompts you to try to understand the situation from the patient's perspective, which in turn helps the patient to feel understood. It also helps you avoid pitfalls that can discourage change, like giving in to your righting reflex by arguing and trying to persuade the person to take insulin.

Evoking

It is easier to provide health care when the people you see with diabetes develop their own ideas into plans for self-care. Of course, this is a collaborative process involving you and the patient. MI centers on helping people accomplish this. The process begins by evoking the patient's ideas of what would work best for him or her. That, in turn, opens up a conversation that explores change by listening reflectively and using open questions, and by elicit–provide–elicit interactions.

The interview in this chapter involves Zoe (see Chapter 8). Her A1c level was 9% at her last appointment. Wanting to avoid insulin, she developed a plan involving a significant increase in physical activity, primarily by playing tennis. She also decided to eat smaller portions of food so that she could lose weight.

In this interview, Zoe is seeing her usual diabetes care provider, a nurse practitioner. The nurse practitioner skillfully avoids persuasion with Zoe. Instead, she carefully guides the conversation by using open questions, reflections, and change rulers (see Chapter 7) to evoke Zoe's own ideas. The nurse practitioner avoids discord (arguments) in the midst of Zoe's constant sustain talk about insulin use during the first half of the conversation.

Insulin Initiation in T2D: An Interview

NURSE PRACTITIONER: Zoe, it's good to see you back. I see you've lost 11 pounds over the past 3 months. (Affirmation) How are you doing?

ZOE: The weight loss feels good. I've been playing tennis 4 days a week, and I'm eating less. I had my A1c done right after I arrived. I'm interested in how it turned out.

NURSE PRACTITIONER: It's 8.7%, compared to 9% 3 months ago. What are your thoughts about it? (Open question that engages Zoe)

ZOE: For all the work I've done, that's not much of a change. My blood glucose tests have shown some values in the 90s and low 100s after tennis. But the levels before breakfast haven't changed much. It's much higher in the early morning than it is after I've just finished an hour of tennis.

NURSE PRACTITIONER: I can see those glucose levels from the download of your meter. Your frustration about the elevated fasting glucose levels is understandable. (Complex reflection) You seem pleased, though, that the levels come down when you exercise. (Complex reflection)

ZOE: When I was here last time, I wanted to be successful taking care of my diabetes. I'm still young [32 years old]. I don't like having diabetes. And the small change in my A1c feels like bad news for me. I don't want to use insulin. Just the idea of it really bothers me. (Sustain talk statements)

NURSE PRACTITIONER: And, of course, using insulin is up to you; I don't make that decision. (Emphasizes personal choice) I wonder, though, if you can see any advantages insulin could offer you. What do you know about this? (Open question that evokes Zoe's knowledge about insulin)

ZOE: I've read about insulin and heard what you've said about it. And I had to use insulin during my pregnancy. It has a big effect on blood glucose levels. I like that part of insulin. (Change talk— desire) But I worry about the low blood glucose levels it could cause. (Sustain talk and some ambivalence about insulin use) And having to take insulin means I didn't succeed.

NURSE PRACTITIONER: You're right about insulin's impact on lowering elevated glucose levels. (Affirmation of Zoe's insight) You've been working to get your A1c down, but now it sounds like you are blaming yourself. Would it be all right with you if I provided some information that might be helpful? (Asking permission before providing information)

ZOE: Yes.

NURSE PRACTITIONER: Diabetes changes over time. This gives you a chance to make decisions about how you want to respond to the changes. (Emphasizes personal preferences) You wanted to re-engage in physical activity and did a great job with that.

(Affirmation) It didn't have the desired effect on your A1c level. As a progressive disease, diabetes gradually makes it harder to manage your glucose without insulin. That's the nature of diabetes, not a failure on your part. Does that make sense?

ZOE: I appreciate what you said about my enjoyment of tennis and all of this not being my fault. Maybe it's my diabetes and not what I'm doing that is causing the high glucose levels. Either way, being in the position of considering insulin is a situation I don't like. (Sustain talk)

NURSE PRACTITIONER: There's no way at all insulin could help you. (Amplified reflection).

ZOE: I didn't say that. I just don't like the situation I'm in. I took insulin when I was pregnant. I did that because I wanted the best outcome for my baby. There are other concerns now. I'm not planning to have another child. Insulin makes people gain weight. I'd like to continue losing weight rather than gaining it. And I would hate having low blood glucose levels when I'm playing tennis. (Sustain talk persists)

NURSE PRACTITIONER: So, one thing you're concerned about with insulin is gaining weight. What might you do to make that less likely? (Evoking Zoe's ideas with an open question)

ZOE: I could continue eating smaller portions and continue the tennis. I might need some help on days I don't play tennis. I tend to snack more on those days.

NURSE PRACTITIONER: How would you go about consuming fewer calories on the days you are not as physically active? (Open questions can make planning easier)

ZOE: I have already started that. I could avoid buying snack foods that I find tempting. (She is already taking steps to lose weight and incorporates those efforts into the plan.)

NURSE PRACTITIONER: You really want to continue losing weight, and you've found a way to avoid tempting snacks.

ZOE: I know I need to do something about my A1c, but I've wanted to avoid insulin for a long time. (Ambivalence)

NURSE PRACTITIONER: You've been doing your best to delay the need for insulin, and also you do see that you need something more. (Double-sided reflection of ambivalence, with change talk last)

ZOE: I'm still young and haven't had diabetes very long. What I'm doing is not having the results I wanted.

NURSE PRACTITIONER: So, on a scale of 0 to 10, how important is it for you to have better control of your blood glucose levels?

ZOE: I know that it's important. That's why I started doing so much about it after I saw you the last time. It's an 8 or 9 in terms of importance.

NURSE PRACTITIONER: So, it's *very* important. You can see that.

ZOE: I just don't know if I can use insulin again.

NURSE PRACTITIONER: I was going to ask you about that too. On the same scale, 0 to 10, how confident are you that you could actually start using insulin again to manage your diabetes?

ZOE: About a 5 or 6.

NURSE PRACTITIONER: Fairly confident! Why 5 or 6 instead of a 1 or 2?

ZOE: I'm saying that not because I want to but because I used insulin when I was pregnant, and it really made a difference.

NURSE PRACTITIONER: It's something you have experience with, and have seen good results before. (Reflection of change talk) What would it take to move your confidence from a 6 to an 8 or 9?

ZOE: I don't want to get low [have hypoglycemia] or have to worry about that when I'm playing tennis.

NURSE PRACTITIONER: I see. You would want to do all you can do to avoid low glucose levels. How might you do that?

ZOE: I'm not sure. When I was pregnant I was not as active as I am now. I didn't have to use insulin when I was exercising.

NURSE PRACTITIONER: Again, it's your decision, but would it be helpful for me to tell you something about what people on insulin can do to avoid hypoglycemia?

ZOE: OK.

NURSE PRACTITIONER: If you decided to take insulin, it would start with taking one dose of basal insulin a day. Basal insulin is helpful for people who have high blood glucose levels when they get up in the morning. You'll also be given a way to adjust the dose of insulin on the days you plan to play tennis. You'd have to test your glucose levels a lot more, four times a day and before and after playing tennis. You can also carry glucose tablets with you to treat lows if they did occur. The pharmacist, who helps people start insulin, and I would be available if you had questions. What are your thoughts about this? (Evoking)

ZOE: It sounds good to vary the insulin based on my blood sugar results and on the days I'm playing tennis. I've used glucose tablets in the past.

NURSE PRACTITIONER: So, this is familiar to you. You already know how to control your weight, and this seems like a realistic way to avoid hypoglycemia.

ZOE: I knew when I came in here today we would talk about insulin. My A1c is not better. That bothers me a lot. What would I have to do to get started on this basal insulin? (Planning continues)

NURSE PRACTITIONER: I would set up appointments for you with a diabetes educator. He's a pharmacist. We work together on insulin starts. You would start with a low dose of insulin. He would also discuss with you how to increase the dose in a way that would make the risk of hypoglycemia lower. The dosing adjustments are small. And you would vary the dose, as I mentioned, on days you are playing tennis. He would also follow up with you to be sure the morning glucose levels are better controlled and you are not having other problems with this. How does that sound?

ZOE: I am willing to try it. I can't say I want to do this, but I really know if I want to stay healthy for myself and my child I need to do something different.

NURSE PRACTITIONER: This is a big step for you. As I think about what you've said today, your family life is something you really value. You worked hard to have a healthy baby when you were pregnant. And being healthy in the future is something you want, even if it involves challenges.

ZOE: I don't like the idea of going on insulin, but I do want to stay healthy.

NURSE PRACTITIONER: It sounds like you are ready to work on this. So, to summarize where we are now . . . you are willing to start using basal insulin, and you will continue playing tennis every other day. You will receive a plan for insulin doses on days you are playing tennis and on days you are not. Your plans for weight control are good ones, and I believe they will work for you. You are going to continue to eat smaller portions and avoid buying unhealthy snacks at the grocery store. Anything else?

ZOE: Just one addition—you told me I could follow up with you if there are any problems.

NURSE PRACTITIONER: That's right. I will make sure with the people out front that you have a way to get timely follow-up with me. And, in any event, I would also like to see you in 2 months.

ZOE: Sounds good.

During the encounter the nurse practitioner evoked change talk as the conversation progressed. In one response to Zoe's frequent sustain talk, the nurse practitioner used an amplified reflection: The reflection ended up eliciting change talk, and the conversation was reframed, "There's no way at all insulin could help you now." Miller and Rollnick (2013, p. 204) describe this as coming alongside. Agreeing in an amplified way with the patient's own sustain talk sometimes evokes change talk. People also seem to enjoy correcting the interviewer's "guess." It ended up changing the conversation. One thing for certain is that agreeing with sustain talk avoids discord; it is the direct opposite of disagreeing with the patient.

> *Agreeing in an amplified way with the patient's own sustain talk sometimes evokes change talk.*

Later in the interview when ambivalence was quite evident, the change rulers were used to strengthen change talk and to facilitate mobilizing change talk. Elicit–provide–elicit was also used to develop a change plan. Patients often need help in developing a plan in this setting because they are unfamiliar with how to begin using insulin. E-P-E fits in well when people exhibit a readiness to consider insulin in their self-care.

The Connection of MI to Diabetes Care

As diabetes progresses over time, people benefit significantly from changing their treatment and self-care. Medications for diabetes have multiplied in recent years, and much more is known about diabetes care (Diabetes Control and Complications Trial Research Group, 1993; UKPDS Study Group, 1998).

Insulin dosing is also now more sophisticated. Little more than two decades ago, there were no clear guidelines for matching insulin dosing with carbohydrate consumption and no formulas for insulin sensitivity factors, a calculation that allows for more accurate insulin dosing when correcting elevated blood glucose levels. Mathematical algorithms with insulin-to-carbohydrate ratios have made it possible to more tightly control glucose levels in the context of meals and snacks, preventing both hyper- and hypoglycemia. These changes in insulin dosing, along with the technologies of self-monitoring of blood glucose values, insulin pumps, and continuous glucose monitoring, have added self-care responsibilities but have also made diabetes easier to control.

However, the benefits of insulin or any other medication or treatment are nil if people do not use them. MI offers a way to address the challenging work facing diabetes practitioners and people with diabetes alike, facilitating self-care options that can improve diabetes outcomes.

Key Points

- Reflective listening begins with concentrating attentively on what is being said, listening for helpful information about the person's motivations and readiness for change.

- Complex reflections begin with a positive statement and then add additional meaning beyond what the client has just said—a guess that adds to what the client may have meant.

- When ambivalence is present, change rulers can be used to strengthen change talk and evoke mobilizing change talk.

- Elicit–provide–elicit interactions help patients who are ready to change. It facilitates their creation of a plan in unfamiliar areas where they may need more information or advice.

CHAPTER 11

Addressing Self-Care during Follow-Up Visits

Diabetes care is a team sport. Unlike acute-care medicine, the long-term management of diabetes is an ongoing process that involves a team of specialists and, most importantly, the patients themselves. No one knows patients as well as they do themselves, so their own expertise is vital when fitting self-care activities into their daily routines.

Fortunately, regular follow-up visits are a routine part of diabetes care, albeit not as often as recommended in many cases. These visits are useful in keeping people in contact with ongoing care and in monitoring their HbA1c levels and other markers of health. They are also an often-missed opportunity for patients to discuss self-care more specifically in order to strengthen their motivation for the marathon run that is diabetes management. It is possible during each follow-up visit to have an MI-based conversation about self-care. MI is not a one-time procedure but rather a clinical style for having ongoing conversations about change.

> *MI is not a one-time procedure but rather a clinical style for having ongoing conversations about change.*

A Progressive Disease Perspective

Because diabetes is a progressive illness, it requires adjustment of both medical and self-care approaches over time. People with T2D may become discouraged when their A1c values continue to climb despite their best efforts. No matter how well patients manage their diet, exercise, self-monitoring, and medication, it is likely that diabetes will continue to progress, though, of course, there are exceptions. Good self-management can slow and even occasionally reverse this progression, but it is important to help patients not despair if A1C continues to increase.

As discussed in the preceding chapter, a common issue with T2D is some patients' dread of having to begin insulin use. With current medications, insulin use can often be delayed, but there comes a point when it is clearly in the patient's best interest to start using it as an alternative to sustained hyperglycemia. Patients need not and should not perceive this as a failure. ("If only I had taken better care of myself!") The focus should be on what is needed *now*, moving forward, to maintain one's health and to prevent future complications. Beginning insulin has some positive aspects and can even be viewed as providing relief (Becker, 2006). It makes glycemic control much easier and dosage can be adjusted according to changes in eating and exercise habits. Once patients begin taking insulin, it is unusual for them to say they want to get off of it.

Raising the Topic

Every follow-up visit is an opportunity to discuss self-care, and most patients are willing to do so if you handle the conversations well. Having taken care of the medical tasks at hand and reviewed lab tests, raising the subject is just a matter of asking an open question:

"So how have you been doing with managing your diabetes?"
"What's going well for you, and what has been more challenging?"
"I wonder if there are any further changes you could make in the interest of your health."

This is also an ideal place to use the bubble sheet shown in Figure 3.1. You can show the person this array of possible subjects for conversation:

"We have a few minutes here to talk about what you're doing to stay healthy. I wonder if there's one of these subjects that you might like to discuss in the time we have left, or perhaps there is another subject you'd prefer to talk about."

The point is to make a conversation about self-care a routine part of each follow-up visit.

Behavioral Review

There are several skills you can use during regular visits with patients that will spur conversation and offer encouragement.

Asking

Beyond asking what the patient would like to discuss, it's also possible for you to ask about particular topics that are important in diabetes management. For example:

> "Tell me a little about how you're getting exercise and staying active."
> "How have you been making decisions about what to eat or not eat?"
> "What's your routine for checking and recording your glucose levels?"
> "How often would you say you miss a dose of metformin?"

Listening

How you respond to information that a patient provides is very important. Often people will offer something that makes them a little vulnerable to see what you'll say:

> INTERVIEWER: How have you been deciding what to eat or not eat? Tell me a bit about that.
>
> PATIENT: I've been doing pretty well in avoiding sweets, though I do have a sweet tooth and sometimes I'll have a dessert.
>
> INTERVIEWER: You've cut down on sweets, and still you enjoy one now and then.
>
> PATIENT: Right! I mean, it's all about moderation, right?
>
> INTERVIEWER: Yes, that's what I'm asking about. How do you decide about what to eat?
>
> PATIENT: Well, I do count carbs like you told me.
>
> INTERVIEWER: You know how to do that. Good.
>
> PATIENT: And someone told me to stay within four carbs per meal, and one per snack.
>
> INTERVIEWER: OK. How's that going?
>
> PATIENT: It's harder when I'm away from home. At home I can read the labels.
>
> INTERVIEWER: It's more challenging when you eat out.
>
> PATIENT: Right. Some menus have carbs on them, but not many.
>
> INTERVIEWER: And how else do you keep track?
>
> PATIENT: I check my sugar level sometimes a couple of hours after a meal, especially if I think I've overdone it. Yesterday I got surprised—it was 228 after lunch.
>
> INTERVIEWER: You don't like it to get that high.

Everything the interviewer did here was either an open question or a reflection. That's a good way to keep a conversation about change moving along. Patients are often concerned that they will be scolded or lectured if they admit to unhealthy behavior. Asking with curiosity and responding with nonjudgmental reflection are skills that build trust and encourage patients to keep speaking with you honestly.

Advising

Nevertheless, it is also feasible for you to offer information or advice, and patients often value this. As discussed in Chapter 6, an MI-consistent way to offer advice or information is *with permission*, and perhaps the most common form of this is when a patient asks you a question. You can even invite such questions:

> "What more would you like to know about taking care of your diabetes?"
> "What else can I tell you that might be helpful?"
> "What have you been wondering about in regard to your diabetes?"

Short of being asked directly, you can *request* permission to introduce a topic:

> "I wonder if we could talk a bit about how exercise affects blood sugar."
> "I could tell you some things that other patients have done to remind them about medications. Would that be of interest?"
> "There's something I'm a little worried about as I look at these results. Can we talk about that?"

Emphasizing Personal Choice

Remember also that it's always the patient who gets to make the decisions about his or her own self-care. Acknowledging this truth can make it more possible for patients to hear what you have to say.

> *It's always the patient who gets to make the decisions about his or her own self-care.*

> "It's really up to you. You're the one who decides what to do."
> "I don't know if this will concern you or not."
> "The fact is that you *can* eat whatever you choose. It's always *your* choice."

Normalizing

Patients are often reluctant to talk about ways in which they have missed medications, "gone off the diet," or "slacked off" on exercise or self-monitoring. The truth is that imperfections are normal, and it's very common for people who start with the best of intentions to gradually drift away from what they know to be in their best interest.

One problem here is what is called the "rule violation effect" (Marlatt & Donovan, 2005), which is often the downfall of New Year's resolutions. With the best of intentions, people set a demanding goal for themselves that is encapsulated in a rule:

"I'm not going to eat sweets."
"I will exercise 5 days a week."
"I'll check my blood sugar 2 hours after every meal."

Then the inevitable happens: they break the rule. Life intervenes, temptation happens, travel disrupts routines. That's not a problem in itself, since it is quite predictable. The problem is in what people then say to themselves after breaking their rule:

"Now I've done it! I'm off my diet."
"I am so weak-willed! I just don't have any self-control."
"What's the point? I guess it's not worth it."
"I'm right back to where I started."

That is the rule violation effect. Telling oneself things like this creates a kind of black-and-white thinking: you're either good or bad, weak or strong. Either you're on your diet or you're off of it. Another destructive idea can accompany such either–or thinking: "Now that I've blown it, now that I'm off my diet, I have nothing to lose. I might as well quit trying." And that kind of thinking has the power to turn a perfectly normal "slip" into a prolonged "relapse" or "failure."

There are two helpful messages to offer when you run into this kind of discouragement. The first is that exceptions are the rule: it is very normal for people to drift away from their best intentions. Second, the key is to get right back on track. If you "fall off the wagon," jump right back on. Self-care is not a contest for perfection; rather, it is a matter of persistence in the long run.

A Case Example

The patient in this case, Adrian, was diagnosed with T2D 5 years earlier and comes back for a routine check-up every 3–4 months. The interviewer in this case is a primary care physician, though it could as easily be a nurse, behavioral health specialist, or diabetes educator.

PHYSICIAN: I have your lab test values, but first I'd like to hear a bit about how you've been doing in managing your diabetes.

Open question

ADRIAN: It's a lot to keep track of.

PHYSICIAN: Indeed, it is—choosing what to eat, testing your sugar levels, using medication, exercising; there's so much that makes a difference. Let me ask you this. Since I saw you last, 3 months ago, would you say you've been doing a little better, about the same, or not quite so well in managing your diabetes?

Reflection

Open question

ADRIAN: I don't know . . .

PHYSICIAN: I promise not to lecture you. What I'd like is to understand what you are experiencing in living with diabetes. So what do you think?

ADRIAN: Maybe not as well.

Offering vulnerability

PHYSICIAN: OK, not quite as well. In what ways? What's been hard?

Reflection and open question

ADRIAN: I haven't been testing my blood very often, and when I do I often don't like what I see.

PHYSICIAN: It's easier just not to think about it.

Reflection

ADRIAN: Well, I do think about it whenever I eat, particularly when I eat things I shouldn't. But I don't like seeing the high numbers.

PHYSICIAN: The numbers somehow make it real.

Reflection

ADRIAN: Yeah, I can't fool the meter. But I know I'm not being as careful as I should about what I eat.

Preparatory change talk

PHYSICIAN: Part of you knows what to do, and another part prefers not to think about it.

Double-sided reflection

ADRIAN: Right! So, what was my A1c level this time?

PHYSICIAN: I'll tell you in a minute, but before I do, let me ask you two questions. First, what will it mean for you if the number is the same as last time or even lower?

ADRIAN: That I've been lucky so far—getting away with being a little careless.

PHYSICIAN: OK. And what will it mean for you if the A1c number has gone up?

Seeking change talk

ADRIAN: That it's time for me to do something different.

Provisional change talk

PHYSICIAN: OK! Well, as you anticipated, it's up a bit: 7.8 this time.

ADRIAN: I was afraid of that.

PHYSICIAN: You had a hunch it was going to be higher.

Reflection

ADRIAN: Yeah, I guess you can't fool the A1c either.

PHYSICIAN: It sounds like you're pretty aware of where you've let things slide and that it's time to step up your efforts a bit. Tell me this. What one change do you think you might make that would help keep your A1c down?

Focusing on positive change and self-efficacy

ADRIAN: When I stop checking my blood level, then I get careless about what I eat.

Change talk

PHYSICIAN: Those two things are tied together for you—eating and checking.

Reflection

ADRIAN: Definitely. If I stop checking, it's like a warning signal, a smoke alarm.

PHYSICIAN: So, one thing you could do is resume testing your sugar levels more often. How might you do that?	*Reflection and open question*
ADRIAN: My numbers in the morning before I eat are usually pretty good. It's the peaks after meals that bother me.	*Change talk*
PHYSICIAN: You don't like seeing how high they are.	*Reflection*
ADRIAN: Well, it just reminds me I'm not eating right. When I checked after lunch yesterday, it was 256. I guess that's a good thing in a way.	*Change talk*
PHYSICIAN: Even though it's bad news, you think it's useful. How so?	*Reflection and open question (asking for elaboration)*
ADRIAN: I don't want high sugar levels, and this is facing up to reality.	*Change talk*
PHYSICIAN: OK. Now, I have a worry here—OK to tell you about it?	*Asking permission*
ADRIAN: Sure.	*Giving permission*
PHYSICIAN: I don't know if this is a concern or not, but, in a way, by the time you test your blood it's already too late to change what you ate, and it sounds like it just makes you feel bad. For most people, feeling bad doesn't help them to change. I wonder what else you could do earlier in addition to checking your glucose level.	*Expressing a concern Giving information Open question*
ADRIAN: What do you suggest?	*Giving permission*
PHYSICIAN: There are quite a few possibilities, and you're the expert on yourself. Here are some things other patients have done that helped them. I don't know if any of these will make sense to you, but see what you think. OK?	*The physician makes a choice here to provide information as requested.*
ADRIAN: OK.	*Giving permission*

PHYSICIAN: One thing we've talked about is writing down everything you eat . . .

ADRIAN: (*interrupting*) That's a real hassle.

PHYSICIAN: OK, as I said, I don't know which of these, if any, might work best for you, but let me just mention some possibilities. So some people have written down whatever they eat before they eat it. Some people count carbohydrates and set a limit per meal. Some find it helpful to keep high-carb foods out of the house. It can also be useful to exercise soon after eating, particularly breakfast or lunch, to burn off some of the carbs. One of my patients who ate out with friends a lot told them he needed to limit carbs and avoid desserts and asked for their support. These are just a few ideas. What sounds like it might work for you?

The physician offers a list of options rather than falling into the trap of presenting one at a time while the patient says what's wrong with it. It facilitates a mental task of choice rather than refutation.

ADRIAN: I know it would be good to avoid buying high-carb junk like potato chips. And I hadn't thought about exercising earlier in the day. My work is flexible enough that I could try that. Usually I've been exercising at night.

Change talk

PHYSICIAN: So, right there are two things that are possible—to avoid high-carb food when you shop or eat out and to move your exercise to earlier in the day. Do you think you'll do those things?

Summary
Asking for commitment language, perhaps too soon

ADRIAN: I'll try.

Activation language, with some doubt about ability

PHYSICIAN: Good! Well, I'll see you again in 3 months, and we can talk about how it's going for you.

With about 5 minutes of conversation the interviewer has been able to elicit a range of change talk and to hone in on possible behavior changes. A plan is emerging that Adrian can try, and the interviewer can check on progress at the next appointment.

Conversations about change have a refreshing side effect: they can ameliorate the stress or fatigue of working with "difficult" patients. People who learn MI remark often about their sense of greater comfort seeing patients who previously seemed to be "difficult"—an attribute that may disappear or at least diminish as your style of conversation changes.

Key Points

- Diabetes is a progressive illness that requires adjustments in medical care and self-care over time.

- Every follow-up visit is an important opportunity to discuss what patients are doing to manage their diabetes and how they might improve their self-care.

- Use open questions and reflections to raise and explore the topic of health behavior change with your patients.

- Imperfection is normal. Help patients avoid the rule violation effect: that once they've "broken" a rule, they have failed, gone "off" their plan, etc.

- When you fall off the wagon, get right back on. This applies to patients (in diet, exercise, and such) as well as clinicians (in the practice of MI).

CHAPTER 12

Substance Use

Ambivalence is common among those who smoke, drink too much, or use illicit drugs. They are usually well aware of the harm or risk associated with their substance use, yet they continue it. This dilemma of "I want it, and I know better" is a familiar one for people with diabetes.

Motivational interviewing was originally developed to help problem drinkers resolve their ambivalence about changing (Miller, 1983). There is extensive clinical trial evidence for the efficacy of MI in helping people reduce or stop substance use. It has been used successfully to treat alcohol, tobacco, and other drug use (Grimshaw & Stanton, 2010; Smedslund et al., 2011; Tait & Hulse, 2003; Vasilaki, Hosier, & Cox, 2006). But, what does all this have to do with diabetes care?

Diabetes and Substance Use

Alcohol use and other drug use are important topics for discussion in diabetes care because they affect so many dimensions of health. Drinking, smoking and illicit drug use were once thought of as specialized issues to be dealt with by referrals, but substance use is increasingly recognized as a primary care concern and one that can often be addressed effectively within routine health care. Substance use disorders are also among the most unrecognized and underaddressed factors that can compromise diabetes care.

Substance use is common in the general population and also among people with diabetes. About 18% of all U.S. adults are binge drinkers (defined as having four or more drinks at a time for women, five or more for men), 30% among those under age 35 (Kanny, Liu, Brewer, & Lu, 2013). About one in four adults smokes tobacco (King, Dube, & Tynan, 2012). Almost one in ten of those over age 12 use illicit drugs, with higher percentages reported among adolescents and young adults. Heavy drinkers (Holbrook, Barrett-Connor, & Wingard, 1990; Howard, Amsten, & Gourevitch, 2004) and smokers (Rimm, Chan, Stampfer, Colditz, & Willett, 1995) are overrepresented among patients with diabetes, although moderate alcohol use appears to lower the risk of developing T2D (Howard et al., 2004; Koppes, Dekker, Hendriks, Bouter, & Heine, 2005).

There are particularly good reasons to attend to these behaviors in diabetes care. Beyond the substantial health risks associated with smoking, heavy drinking, and illicit drug use, substance use poses special risks for people with diabetes. Alcohol, for example, blocks the liver's ability to produce glycogen and to break it down into glucose, increasing the risk of hypoglycemia—an effect that can endure for hours after drinking. Given the sedative effects of alcohol as a central nervous system depressant, there is danger of falling asleep with plummeting blood sugar levels. Drug use more generally may cause people to overlook the signs of hypoglycemia, to neglect glucose monitoring, and to skip meals or needed medications. Stimulants can spike blood sugar. Negligence in self-care can be exacerbated by impairment of short-term memory, and by the enhancing (marijuana) or suppressing (cocaine, stimulants) effects of drugs on appetite.

Substance use poses special risks for people with diabetes.

The risks of tobacco use are well known, and, again, are multiplied for people with diabetes. Smoking can decrease insulin absorption and influence glucose tolerance tests. Vasoconstriction increases risk of damage to the eyes and kidneys and can exacerbate neuropathy and sexual dysfunction. Smokers have higher rates of hypertension, heart disease, and stroke—cardiovascular risks that are already elevated with diabetes—and smoking dramatically increases risk for limb amputation.

Asking Patients about Substance Use

Until it becomes routine practice, patients coming for diabetes care may not expect to be asked about their substance use. Consider this as part of routine care, and soon your patients will see it that way as well.

Raising a Sensitive Topic

You need to know about your patients' substance use. We recommend raising the subject as a routine topic, one that you need to know about in helping people manage their health. If you feel comfortable in asking these questions, your patients are more likely to feel at ease in responding honestly. During a diabetes consultation it may be helpful to preface these potentially sensitive questions with something like this:

"There are a few questions that I ask all of my patients about things that can really affect your health when you have diabetes. Would it be all right to take a few minutes to talk about these now?"

A simple preface like this normalizes the questions ("I ask all of my patients"), highlights their importance in diabetes care, and asks permission. It can be useful to intermix the substance use questions as part of a broader screening for risk and protective factors such as diet and exercise, stress, and depression.

Screening Questions

With regard to smoking, it has been routine in health care to ask simply, "Do you smoke?" Such a closed yes/no question is less suitable, however, when asking about alcohol and other drugs, and it is also less likely to get at the whole truth. A "Yes" answer to "Do you drink alcohol?" still tells you relatively little. The occasional glass of wine is of less concern than heavier drinking that significantly increases blood alcohol concentration (BAC). We recommend this screening question for men:

> "How many times in the past year have you had four or more drinks in a day?"

and for women:

> "How many times in the past year have you had three or more drinks in a day?"

The cutoff point is lower for females because women tend to be smaller than men. Also, men metabolize alcohol in the stomach more quickly before it gets to the bloodstream; so, even at the same body mass, a man will have a lower BAC than a woman drinking the same amount of alcohol (Miller & Muñoz, 2013).

Patients may have a very liberal idea of what constitutes "one drink." A woman told us that she only had two drinks a day, but her "drink" was an 8-ounce tumbler of gin topped with a thin layer of vermouth. Use a simple card like the one shown in Figure 12.1 with patients. All of the drinks described there contain the same amount of the same kind of alcohol (ethanol). Here is how you might use a card like this in the screening process.

CLINICIAN: Now, I'd like to ask you about your alcohol use. Have you had any drink containing alcohol in the past year?

PATIENT: Yes.

> Each of the drinks below contains about the same amount of alcohol.
>
> 12 ounces of   beer   (5% alcohol)
>
> 5 ounces of   table wine   (12% alcohol)
>
> 1.5 ounces of   liquor   (40% alcohol)

FIGURE 12.1. What is "one drink"?

CLINICIAN: OK. Now, here's what I mean when I say "one drink." All of these drinks contain the same amount of alcohol: about 12 ounces of beer, or 5 ounces of wine, or an ounce-and-a-half of hard liquor. In the past year how many times have you had three [for women; four for men] or more drinks like this in 1 day?

PATIENT: Oh, not very often. Once a month, maybe.

CLINICIAN: So, 12 times in a year, perhaps.

PATIENT: Or a few more.

CLINICIAN: OK, thanks. And on a typical day when you do have some alcohol, how many drinks do you usually have?

PATIENT: Well, I don't drink that often, but maybe two or three glasses of wine.

The point is not to pin down exactly how much your patient is drinking or to make a diagnosis but simply to decide whether you should have a conversation (as described later in this chapter) about alcohol and diabetes. For nondrinkers, you can simply say, "Good! Alcohol use can be tricky for people with diabetes, so that's a good choice."

In asking about illicit drug use, an effective screening question (Smith, Schmidt, Allensworth-Davies, & Saitz, 2010) is:

"How many times in the past year have you used an illegal drug or used a prescription medication for nonmedical reasons?"

If the answer is greater than "0," a simple follow-up is "Tell me a bit more about that," and then use reflective listening (rather than closed questions) to learn more. For example:

CLINICIAN: Now, let me ask you this: How many times in the past year have you used an illegal drug or used a prescription medication for nonmedical reasons?

PATIENT: A few times, I guess.

CLINICIAN: Tell me a bit more about that.

PATIENT: Well, I've used cocaine a few times.

CLINICIAN: So, that's one thing you've used. (Reflection)

PATIENT: And marijuana, of course.

CLINICIAN: OK. What else?

PATIENT: I had some dental work done, and she gave me some pain medicine. Does that count?

CLINICIAN: Tell me about your experience with that.

PATIENT: I had a tooth pulled, and it helped with the pain afterward. I kept them around in the medicine cabinet, and I take one or two now and then.

CLINICIAN: You've liked how it feels when you take one. (Reflection)

PATIENT: Sometimes, yes.

To have an honest conversation, it is important not to jump right in with concern or advice (though that's what your righting reflex may tell you to do). There is time for this later. Reflective listening allows the patient to talk to you comfortably without feeling judged or criticized.

Talking with Patients about Substance Use

The purpose of the screening questions above is to determine whether further conversation about substance use is warranted. In the context of diabetes care, your concern is with how the substance use may affect glycemic control and patient self-care. When a conversation is warranted, there are three components to keep in mind:

1. Express your concern.
2. Explain the reasons for your concern by providing relevant information.
3. Explore what behavior changes the patient might make in the interest of self-care.

Avoid switching into a lecture mode! It should be a conversation, with ample amounts of listening as well as sharing your expertise. There is solid evidence that a brief intervention of this kind within the context of health care often prompts a significant change in substance use (e.g., Babor et al., 2007; Bernstein et al., 2005; Grimshaw & Stanton, 2010; Smedslund et al., 2011).

Express Your Concern

The elicit–provide–elicit method is particularly useful here.

A good first step is to ask what your patient already knows about the topic of concern. Telling patients what they already know is not helpful, whereas having the patient voice the risks is a form of change talk.

CLINICIAN: I wonder what you know about the risks of smoking in general, and for people with diabetes in particular.	*Elicit*
ROBIN: Well, I know it's bad for your heart.	*Change talk*
CLINICIAN: In what way?	*Elicit—asking for more change talk, not just agreeing*
ROBIN: Doesn't it increase blood pressure or something, and make you more likely to have a heart attack?	*Change talk*
CLINICIAN: Yes, that's right, it does. And how about circulation?	*Provide* *Elicit*
ROBIN: Oh, yeah. It cuts off circulation, I think.	*Change talk*
CLINICIAN: Right! It reduces blood flow to your hands and feet, for example. Can you see why that's especially risky for people with diabetes?	*Provide* *Elicit*
ROBIN: Not really. Is it?	*Giving permission for information*
CLINICIAN: Yes, definitely. Higher glucose makes your blood more thick and sticky, and that impairs blood supply to your extremities, your eyes . . .	*Provide*
ROBIN: My eyes, too?	*Giving permission for information*
CLINICIAN: Uh-huh. That's why it's good to have your eyes checked regularly. And that's why I always check your feet, to see how your circulation and sensation are there. Does that make sense to you?	*Provide* *Elicit*

ROBIN: I guess so. I know people with   *Change talk*
diabetes sometimes have a leg ampu-
tated.

CLINICIAN: It's a risk. And when you   *Provide*
smoke . . . (*pause*)   *Elicit*

ROBIN: It makes it worse.   *Change talk*

CLINICIAN: Yes, it does. People with dia-   *Provide*
betes who smoke are about twice as
likely to suffer an amputation or lose
their eyesight.

ROBIN: I see.

CLINICIAN: So, that's one reason I'm very   *Provide*
concerned about your smoking. Does   *Elicit*
that make sense?

ROBIN: Yes.

Notice that E-P-E is essentially a Socratic approach, starting with what the patient already knows and providing small pieces of additional information to enhance his or her motivation to change. It helps patients reach their own conclusion rather than just hearing it from you. When the elicit–provide–elicit process works well, patients literally talk themselves into changing.

> *When the elicit–provide–elicit process works well, patients literally talk themselves into changing.*

It is fine to express your specific concern for patients' health and welfare, even (and particularly) if they themselves don't understand the problem, but don't launch into lecturing and ordering ("You can't smoke when you have diabetes!"). It is always the patients who get to choose what they will do, and the goal of your conversation is to help them make healthy choices. People respond much better to concern than to criticism or scare tactics. Express your concern and ask permission to have the conversation, honoring the patient's autonomy.

> "I want to tell you that, as your doctor, I am really worried about your health and how smoking affects your diabetes. I'm not going to lecture you, but I wonder if it would be OK for us to talk about that for a bit."

> "Based on what I know about diabetes, I'm a little concerned about the drinking that you describe. What you decide to do is up to you, but I'd like for us to talk a bit about how alcohol can affect your diabetes. Would that be all right?"

"Many people who smoke marijuana think of it as a very safe drug. I wonder what you know about how it interacts with diabetes and self-care. Could you tell me a bit about that?"

Explain Your Concern

Sometimes asking what patients already know doesn't yield much information. It may never have occurred to them that there is a connection between substance use and diabetes self-care. Providing relevant information is important, and it can be done well with an E-P-E approach.

CLINICIAN: So, you really don't see why alcohol is something you should be careful about . . .	*With this kind of reflection, it is particularly important to inflect your voice downward at the end, making it a statement. An upward inflection at the end turns it into a potentially accusatory question.*
DALE: That's right. I'm not an alcoholic or anything.	*Sustain talk*
CLINICIAN: And I'm certainly not implying that you are. It's the effect of alcohol on diabetes that worries me. May I give you a little information to consider? What you do with it is up to you.	*Asking permission* *Respecting autonomy*
DALE: Sure.	
CLINICIAN: There are actually several things that can happen to drinkers with diabetes. One is blood sugar getting too low. Alcohol keeps your liver from producing a normal amount of sugar—so, it can be easy to take too much insulin and wind up in insulin shock. You look a little confused. How can I explain it better?	*Provide* *Elicit*
DALE: I just didn't know that alcohol lowers your sugar level.	
CLINICIAN: Oh! Yes, it can; so, it makes insulin dosing more unpredictable.	*Provide*

And you should test often if you're drinking. Can you see why?	*Elicit*

DALE: I guess it's a double whammy.

CLINICIAN: Insulin and alcohol, right. And alcohol can also make you drowsy. It's a sedative. Does that ever happen to you when you drink?	*Provide* *Elicit*

DALE: Sure—after I have a few drinks.

CLINICIAN: So, you're more likely to fall asleep, maybe with dropping blood sugar. And that's . . . (*slight pause*)	*Provide* *Elicit*

DALE: Not good.	*Change talk*

CLINICIAN: Indeed. May I tell you one more thing that often happens sometimes?	*Asking permission*

DALE: OK.

CLINICIAN: I don't know if this applies to you, but often when people drink they kick back and don't pay as much attention to what they're doing.	*Provide*

DALE: I chill out.

CLINICIAN: And that means you may pay less attention to what you're eating, how much you're drinking, testing your sugar, how much insulin you're taking. In other words, you can get a little careless. Does that ever happen?	*Provide* *Elicit*

DALE: Sometimes, yeah.

CLINICIAN: So, there's a triple whammy— three things alcohol does. Can you tell me all three?	*Provide* *Elicit*

DALE: Getting sleepy, lower sugar, not paying as much attention.

CLINICIAN: Exactly.

DALE: So, are you saying I shouldn't drink at all?

CLINICIAN: Well, let's talk a little about what you might do with this . . .

Explore Behavior Change

So, you have expressed and explained your concern. Don't stop there! A moment when the reasons for concern are more salient is a window of opportunity. If all you do is raise anxiety without exploring what patients can do, you haven't done them any favor.

The next step, then, is to discuss what changes the patient might make in the interest of health but avoid stepping into the expert role here and telling the patient what to do. People are the experts on their own lives and behavior, so the process of behavior change is one of negotiation, not prescription. If a patient asks for suggestions, you can certainly offer them—preferably a menu of options. You can also ask the patient's permission to share some possibilities.

The two most common forms of substance use are smoking and drinking. With smoking, of course, the healthiest option is to quit altogether. Here you can offer whatever smoking cessation aids or programs are available in your clinic or community. Why do we suggest offering patients a menu of options instead of one at a time? Here's why:

PATIENT: Well, how do people quit smoking?

CLINICIAN: There are several options. Some people just go cold turkey.

PATIENT: I've heard you go crazy for the first week or so, that the withdrawal is really bad.

CLINICIAN: OK. Well, there's the nicotine patch or gum, and there are other medications that can help with withdrawal.

PATIENT: I don't want to take any drugs. Too many side effects, and you can get hooked on the gum.

CLINICIAN: The American Cancer Society offers good groups to help people quit.

PATIENT: I don't like talking to a group of strangers.

With the "How about this one?" approach, you can wind right back up arguing for change while the patient tells you what's wrong with each option. A better strategy is to present a range of options and ask the patient which seems like a good place to start:

PATIENT: Well, how do people quit smoking?

CLINICIAN: I can tell you some things that other patients have done successfully. Would that be of interest?

PATIENT: OK.

CLINICIAN: I'll describe a variety of options, and so listen and then tell me which of these might make the most sense for you. I think people have good hunches about what is likely to work for them.

PATIENT: All right.

CLINICIAN: Actually, the most common one is just going cold turkey. Some people cut down by half or so before they quit, and others just do it. Then there are different medications that some people have found helpful. Some help you taper off of nicotine, and others help with craving. There are free groups available to prepare and learn strategies to quit, and there are individual professionals who specialize in this. There are also some good websites or books I could recommend. Some people tell their friends they are quitting and ask for their support. It just depends on how much help you want along the way. Which of these do you think might be the best approach for you, given what you know about yourself? Or maybe you have other good ideas of what would work for you.

With regard to alcohol, some people find it easiest to quit drinking altogether. For others, moderation is the key. Truly moderate drinking is not a risk factor with diabetes. People who have been heavier or more dependent drinkers, though, may have a harder time maintaining moderation (Miller & Muñoz, 2013). For those with diabetes who do choose to use alcohol, Figure 12.2 contains some practical safety guidelines.

CLINCIAN: So, you see why I'm worried about the amount that you drink sometimes. What are you thinking about that at this point? *Elicit*

DALE: I don't really want to give it up completely.

CLINICIAN: That leaves a couple of options: continuing as you have been or cutting down some. What do you think about that? *Provide*

Elicit

DALE: I'm willing to think about cutting down, I guess. *Mobilizing change talk*

CLINICIAN: Let me show you this sheet of ideas from the American Diabetes Association for people who drink. Tell me what you think about each one of these. *Provide: Clinician presents the list in Figure 12.2.*

Elicit

If you plan to drink, here are some things you can do to protect yourself:
- Don't drink on an empty stomach. Eat something before and while drinking.
- The dangers of drinking with diabetes are related to *how much* you drink. Limit yourself to one drink per day for women and or two drinks per day for men (12 oz. of beer, 5 oz. of wine, or 1.5 oz. of distilled spirits).
- Avoid drink mixes that contain sugar.
- Test your blood glucose frequently, and especially often if you are also exercising or dancing.
- Always wear your medical ID.
- Sip your drink slowly. Spread it out over time, and switch to a nonalcohol, nonsugar drink.
- Mix and pour your own drink so that you know what it contains.
- To avoid sleeping with hypoglycemia, set an alarm to check your blood glucose during the night after drinking.
- Drink with someone who is aware you have diabetes and knows how to treat low blood glucose.
- Never drink and drive.

FIGURE 12.2. Safety guidelines for alcohol use and diabetes. Based on American Diabetes Association guidelines.

DALE: Well, I don't usually drink on an empty stomach. It's usually wine with dinner or afterward.

CLINICIAN: OK. So, that's one good thing. What else?

DALE: And I don't like sweet drinks. I know the sugar is bad for me.

CLINICIAN: All right.

DALE: Now, one drink a day. I drink more than that.

CLINICIAN: That would be a big reduction for you. *Reflection*

DALE: Yes. I'll have a whole bottle of wine sometimes.

CLINICIAN: And, given what you know now, what do you think about this? *Elicit (suppressing the righting reflex)*

DALE: I guess I should cut down. I can try it. *Change talk*

CLINICIAN: Good! I have some information here to help if you want it.

*Provide (e.g., National
Institute on Alcohol Abuse
and Alcoholism, 1996)*

DALE: OK. So, let's see: I don't drink and
drive.

CLINICIAN: Not at all.

*A reflection, but an implied
question*

DALE: No, I just have wine at home.

CLINICIAN: All right. How about some of
the other ideas on this list?

Elicit

Note that, instead of just handing the patient the information sheet, the clinician spends a few minutes considering options on the list and eliciting change talk. Later on, at the end of the session, the clinician might offer a summary something like this:

CLINICIAN: You seem to understand the
risks of heavier drinking for people
with diabetes—falling blood sugar,
not paying attention to self-care,
falling asleep. That's good. Let me
see if I understand what you plan
to do, then. You said you want to
cut back on the amount of wine you
have, down to a glass or two per
night. I think that's a very good idea.
You liked the idea of sipping more
slowly and putting the glass down in
between sips. I gave you the booklet
with some other ideas for you to read.
You plan to start wearing a medical alert, and you said you would be
careful to check your glucose more
often when you drink. And if you go
over your limit of one or two glasses,
you would set your alarm to check
again during the night. Is that right?

*Collecting Dale's change
talk into a summary*

DALE: Yes.

CLINICIAN: Well, let me ask you this: On
a scale from 0 to 10, where 0 is not at
all important and 10 is extremely

important, how important would you
say it is for you to do these things
you've mentioned?

DALE: Seven or eight.

CLINICIAN: Really high! You hadn't
thought much about all this before,
but now that you have, you see that
it's important. Why such a high
number?

DALE: I just hadn't thought about alcohol
and insulin being a double whammy.

CLINICIAN: You want to be careful.   *Reflection—continuing the*
                                                       paragraph

DALE: Yes.   *Change talk*

CLINICIAN: So, that's why it's important
to you to do what you've talked
about. How confident are you that
you can do these things? Zero to ten.

DALE: Eight.

CLINICIAN: Eight again. Pretty sure that
you'll take these steps to protect
yourself.

DALE: Yes, I want to.   *Change talk, though still*
                                                       preparatory

CLINICIAN: Will you try this, then?   *Asking at an activation, not*
                                                       a commitment, level

DALE: Yes, I will.

CLINICIAN: Great! Well, I'll see you again
in 3 months, and we can talk about
how it's going. And, if there is anything I can do to help you make these
changes in the meantime, just call the
office or send me an e-mail. OK?

DALE: OK. Thanks.

In this case, the conversation got all the way to a specific change plan
and mobilizing change talk. Not every brief consultation about behavior
change gets that far, of course, but this kind of conversation is far more
likely to trigger change than is just dispensing uninvited information and
advice.

Follow Up

Changing a well-established habit usually takes more than one try. Mark Twain once quipped, "Giving up smoking is the easiest thing in the world. I know because I've done it thousands of times." Don't be discouraged if your first conversation about change isn't sufficient. Place an alert in patients' charts or use a tickler file to check back with them about their substance use when they visit. Keep notes on what motivations they expressed and what steps they had planned to take, and ask what has happened since your last visit.

If there has been no change, revisit the steps above: explore the patient's own knowledge and motivations for change, renew your own concern, and ask what steps the person is willing to take before your next visit.

Sometimes patients will express shame, guilt, or hopelessness when there has been no change. These hinder rather than encourage future change efforts. Feeling bad about themselves doesn't usually help people to change. Here is another place where you can make a difference.

DALE: I know I said I would try to quit, but I didn't do it. I'm sorry to disappoint you.

CLINICIAN: Oh, this isn't a change you would make for my benefit. What I'm concerned about is how this affects your diabetes and your health more generally. What do you remember about our conversation as to why smoking is especially dangerous with diabetes?

DALE: It was something about circulation and my eyes.

CLINICIAN: That's right. Smoking causes your blood vessels to constrict, reducing blood flow to important places like your eyes, your hands, and feet. And diabetes also reduces blood supply. Do you remember?

DALE: Yes, the double whammy. I did quit for a week, but then I went right back to smoking.

CLINICIAN: Wow! How did you manage to quit for a week? You've been smoking for a long time.

DALE: It was right after I saw you last time. It was really hard.

CLINICIAN: But you made it for a week. That's encouraging. So, you were trying the cold turkey way, toughing it out on your own.

DALE: Yeah. I like doing things myself.

CLINICIAN: And lots of people do quit smoking on their own. Other people find it's helpful to have some support, as we discussed last time.

DALE: I just don't think I can do it.

CLINICIAN: It seems like it's just impossible—too hard for you. (Amplified reflection)

DALE: Well, not impossible, but I've tried several times and always went back.

CLINICIAN: So, your experience is like many other patients I've seen. Smokers usually try several times before they finally quit, often as many as seven times or more. Are you willing to try again?

DALE: Maybe.

CLINICIAN: And what about having a bit of help on this round? It's up to you. Can we talk about some options?

DALE: OK.

Affirming Progress

With addictive behaviors like substance use, people often get stuck in perfectionism: Either you are 100% successful or you've failed. That kind of all-or-none thinking can actually get in the way of progress.

> "I blew it! I was going to stay away from alcohol and now I've had a drink."
> "Now I've done it! I'm off my diet."
> "I relapsed! I'm never going to be able to quit smoking."

You can help to counteract this negative thinking by affirming every positive step that your patient *does* make in the direction of change. To be sure, there are individuals who decide to quit and do it once and for all. A common pattern in recovery from alcohol dependence is that episodes of drinking grow shorter and less severe and are separated by longer periods of abstinence (Miller, 1996).

Illicit Drug Use

Thus far, we have focused primarily on alcohol and tobacco, the most commonly used drugs that complicate diabetes care. As discussed at the beginning of this chapter, however, the use of other drugs can similarly compromise self-care and dysregulate blood glucose. The National Institute on Drug Abuse (2010) recommends routinely asking about drug use in health care consultations, and there are particularly good reasons for doing so in the management of diabetes. Even the single screening question suggested earlier in this chapter is a big improvement over ignoring other drug use.

Conversations about illicit drug use need not be different in form from those described above. Brief health care–based interventions grounded in

MI have been reported to reduce the use of drugs including marijuana, cocaine, and heroin (e.g., Bernstein et al., 2005, 2009; D'Amico, Miles, Stern, & Meredith, 2008). Of course, referral to specialist treatment is also an option when less intensive interventions have not yielded change (e.g., Sobell & Sobell, 2000).

Key Points

- Alcohol, tobacco, and other drug use can seriously dysregulate blood glucose and compromise diabetes management.
- Therefore screening for these forms of substance use is appropriate in diabetes care.
- Some simple single questions can be used to screen for alcohol and other drug use concerns.
- MI was originally developed to address addictive behaviors, and an MI-based conversation about change can impact your patient's substance use.
- Elicit–provide–elicit remains a useful approach for offering your patient important information.
- Three key steps in a conversation about substance use and diabetes are:
  1. Express your concern.
  2. Explain the reasons for your concern by providing relevant information.
  3. Explore what behavior changes the patient might make in the interest of self-care.

CHAPTER 13

Psychological Stress
and Depression

This chapter deals with two common obstacles to self-care, psychological distress and depression. There is a bidirectional relationship between diabetes and both of these mental health conditions. Research suggests that people who have chronic distress also have higher risks of developing diabetes, and diabetes by itself can lead to distress (Pouwer, Kupper, & Adriaanse, 2010). The same bidirectional relationship is true of depression. People with depression have higher risks of developing diabetes (Golden et al., 2008), and people with diabetes who are free of depression have a twofold higher risk of developing it as compared to people without diabetes (Anderson, Freedland, Clouse, & Lustman, 2001; Katon, 2009) .

Peyrot and Rubin found that psychological distress and depression occur twice as frequently among women than men and that unmarried individuals have higher rates of depression than married ones. Depression occurs most frequently in the 40–49 age group, whereas distress is most frequent among those in their 30s. People with college degrees have half the risk of depression or distress as those who did not finish high school (Peyrot & Rubin, 1997). Obesity alone and chronic diabetic complications (e.g., retinopathy, end-stage kidney disease, lower limb amputations) both carry higher risks of depression (Dragan & Akhtar-Danesh, 2007; Hedayati, Minhajuddin, Toto, Morris, & Rush, 2009).

In this chapter, we discuss the use of MI in screening people for distress or depression and in discussions focusing on referrals to mental health professionals. Both psychological stress and depression are easily overlooked in diabetes care (Li et al., 2010). This does not mean that care providers are unconcerned about whether or not their patients have these conditions. It relates more to the fact that when people are distressed or depressed their diabetes self-care becomes compromised, often leading to serious complications. Medical and nursing professionals focus on the diabetes, and when self-care appears to be diminishing, an intense focus on uncontrolled diabetes can displace attention directed toward mental health issues. Yet, attending to distress and depression with uncontrolled diabetes can improve diabetes-related health care outcomes.

Psychological Distress in Diabetes

Distress is unpleasant and yet very common. It can accompany discrete events, like the challenges of completing a difficult work project or preparing for a test. Once the task is completed, the distress usually resolves itself. It can also recur frequently, however, as when working through difficulties with friends, family members, or work supervisors. Distress caused by having chronic conditions like diabetes takes on a continuous dimension. In contrast to common episodic distress, people with diabetes experience the physical and emotional presence of something that does not go away, something most people do not have and something that requires difficult self-care (see Table 13.1).

> *In contrast to common episodic distress, people with diabetes experience the physical and emotional presence of something that does not go away, something most people do not have and something that requires difficult self-care.*

Health care practitioners are aware of the obvious stresses associated with diabetes when people are first diagnosed or when complications develop. Sometimes, however, the ongoing stress is less obvious. People with diabetes often have to think about diabetic problems on a daily basis. Here are just a few of their typical day-to-day thoughts:

"I hope the amount of insulin I took at lunchtime works today. I'm so tired of having high glucose levels before supper . . . but it's hell to be low at work anytime!"

"I just ate breakfast like they told me to, but I always feel starved when I do that."

"It's so expensive to take care of my diabetes. Sometimes I don't have enough money left over for my family. Somehow this has to change."

"I couldn't get my diabetes under control. So, I decided to just stop doing the blood glucose tests—they're always high anyway."

"I wish I could live and eat anything that I want the same way everyone else does."

"I don't like telling people I have diabetes"

TABLE 13.1. Day-to-Day Tasks of Having Diabetes and Providing Self-Care

Self-care tasks	T2D	T1D
Diabetes medication(s)	• One to four oral diabetes drugs or • Insulin injection(s) and two to three oral diabetes drugs or • Insulin by injection or insulin plus metformin orally	• Insulin administered by injections or by insulin pump therapy
Preventive medications and/or common medications (for BP)	• Statins (lower LDL cholesterol levels) • ACE or ARB (for treating hypertension and for the prevention/treatment of retinopathy or kidney disease) • Aspirin: none if < 5% risk for CVD; use is recommended with risk for CVD > 10% and for all men > 50 years old and women > 60 years old (if tolerated)	• Statin starting at 40 years old for people with increased cardiovascular risk or LDL > 100 mg/dl • ACE or ARB (drug treatment for hypertension, diabetic kidney disease, and/or retinopathy) • Aspirin: none if < 5% risk for CVD; use is recommended with risk for CVD > 10% and for all men > 50 years old and women > 60 years old (if tolerated)
Medical follow-up for diabetes	Quarterly, more frequently if problems or complications	Quarterly, more frequently if problems or complications
Dental care	Twice annually	Twice annually
Screening for retinopathy	Annual screening or visits more often for treating retinopathy	Annual screening or visits more often for treating retinopathy
Healthy eating recommendations	Every day, in coordination with medications; if on intensive insulin therapy, it is necessary to accurately count the grams of carbohydrates and then provide an appropriate dose of insulin for every meal and snack	Every day, with the need to accurately count the grams of carbohydrate and then provide an appropriate dose of insulin for every meal and snack (T1D requires intensive insulin therapy)
Self-monitoring of blood glucose levels	• One to seven times weekly if taking oral medications • Four more times daily if on insulin	Four to 10 times daily

(continued)

TABLE 13.1. (continued)

Foot self-examinations	Daily if loss of protective sensation (indicative of diabetic sensory neuropathy) or PAD.	Daily if loss of protective sensation (indicative of diabetic sensory neuropathy) or PAD.
Physical activity	ADA standards of care advise 150 minutes weekly of moderately vigorous aerobic activity	ADA standards of care advise 150 minutes weekly of moderately vigorous aerobic activity
A plan for managing acute illnesses or stress	Yes	Yes
Substantially increased lifelong expenses	Diabetes medications are the most costly ones in nonspecialty care (Weinstein, 2014)	In addition to high costs for insulin, people with T1D often have increased expenses for insulin pumps and related supplies and CGM and its related supplies
Other	With the risk of hypoglycemia when using insulin, it is helpful to inform friends and coworkers of its symptoms and treatment	With the risk of hypoglycemia when using insulin, it is helpful to inform friends and coworkers of its symptoms and treatment

Notes. ACE, angiotensin-converting enzyme; ADA, American Diabetes Association; ARB, angiotensin receptor blocker; BP, blood pressure; CGM, continuous glucose monitoring; CVD, cardiovascular disease; LDL, low-density lipoprotein; PAD, peripheral arterial disease.

These background thoughts are frequently present, but people rarely use them as openers during their diabetes appointments with you. Instead, patients often avoid bringing up distress or dismiss it as unimportant. Others have become inured to the presence of uncontrolled diabetes and can even seem relaxed and flippant about their need for improving self-care. One obese patient commented, "My blood sugar hasn't been under 200 for years!" Even when distress is addressed, there remains the overriding reality that this disease can cause serious complications and shorten life. This information becomes a weighty burden.

Life with diabetes is also challenging. Conscientious efforts to manage glucose levels may not result in hitting the targets of good control. Keeping up with the tasks of self-care (see Table 13.1) is tiring. The stress of managing diabetes and getting a mix of desired and undesired results is so frustrating that it can lead people to put aside conscientious self-care efforts even though doing so becomes yet another source of distress. People with uncontrolled diabetes frequently say that they *truly desire* to control their diabetes, but many of life's distractions and hardships deflect that commitment.

Diabetes can go awry when a person is stressed. Blood glucose levels rise, and self-care can be compromised (Ogbera & Adeyemi-Doro, 2011). Glycogenic hormones, especially cortisol and catecholamines, are secreted in response to stress, elevating blood glucose levels and making diabetes even more difficult to control.

In responding to patients with psychological distress, it is helpful to attend to styles for coping and social support rather than just addressing the diabetes problems. This creates a strong case for the value of mental health professionals on diabetes treatment teams. Of course, approaches based solely on psychosocial treatment are helpful but may not correct the metabolic control of diabetes (Karlsen, Oftedal, & Bru, 2012).

It is important to find out if a patient is experiencing distress. People at times deny they have it. It may only become apparent when family members accompany a person to his or her diabetes appointments because of concerns about stress experienced by them and/or the family member with diabetes. Unless you ask about distress, it is likely to be dismissed and remain masked as just another example of inadequate self-care.

Telling all your patients you ask regularly about the distresses of having diabetes lets them know you have interests and concerns about the impacts it has on them. It opens up conversations about a sensitive topic: "I like to ask all my patients about stress because it occurs often in life and in diabetes self-care too. What sorts of stress do you have with your diabetes or in other areas of your life?" Even if diabetes is not the source of distress, problems in other life areas impact glycemic control and overall perceptions of wellness.

The following interview focuses on Rosa, a woman with insulin-requiring T2D. She was diagnosed 6 years earlier. Her A1c has increased over the past 3 months. She is married and has three children, ages 11 to 18. She is seeing a physician whose practice is limited to people with diabetes.

PHYSICIAN: It's good to see you today. How have things been going for you? (Nonfocused open question)

ROSA: I'm doing OK. I've had a few more high glucoses.

PHYSICIAN: Your blood glucose has been more difficult for you to control (Complex reflection).

ROSA: Yeah. I bet you can see that from my A1c. It'll be higher.

PHYSICIAN: It's gone up—from 7.4% last time to 8.8% now. What do you think about that? (Evoking)

ROSA: I backed off of my insulin some. I've had a lot going on.

PHYSICIAN: You've had a lot going on and it's affected your diabetes.

Diabetes is hard to take care of. You likely recall that I ask all my patients about stress. (A segue to screening for distress) I'm wondering about that now.

ROSA: My husband got cut back at work right after I last saw you. He's working about half-time, and it's put a big burden on me. I'm trying to pick up extra shifts at the hospital whenever I can. We're struggling.

PHYSICIAN: You feel stressed out; that's caused glucose levels to go up. But you're also not taking your insulin all the time. (Shifts discussion to the patient's focus on her insulin)

ROSA: You're close to something I don't like talking about. Only my husband knows this. . . . (20- to 30-second pause) We just don't have enough money to pay for things. My kids are getting older and they are more expensive now than when they were little. My husband's looking for more work. I get some overtime from work. But the insulin I'm using is really expensive. It's early in the year. I haven't met my deductible (insurance deductible). I have to spread insulin out. I'm still taking the long-acting one. But the mealtime doses are cut back, and sometimes I skip the lunchtime doses.

PHYSICIAN: You're having a rough time. You're working hard and are really concerned about your family. It's a difficult situation. I can understand how you'd feel distressed. (Reflections expressing empathy)

ROSA: We've always gotten by, but not by much. Losing his income has both of us stressed out. There are a few more arguments between me and my husband. But we still care a lot for each other. We make up.

PHYSICIAN: You are doing everything you can to make more income. What else do you think would help? (Evoking Rosa's ideas)

ROSA: Are there any cheaper drugs for my diabetes?

PHYSICIAN: You're taking brand name insulins that are newer. There are generic insulins—Regular insulin, that's short-acting, and NPH, a longer-acting one. We would have to change the doses on them. They are about half the price.

ROSA: That's a big difference. Why am I on the expensive ones?

PHYSICIAN: The insulins you are on are new and are modified to become activated more rapidly or for longer periods of time. That's why we'd have to modify the doses. NPH and Regular insulins have been used for many, many years. We can do that. What do you think? (Evoking)

ROSA: It would save money. I'd be willing to try them if they're safe.

PHYSICIAN: All insulin has the risk of causing hypoglycemia. Some say it's more common with NPH or Regular. But I think we can get around that by starting them at low doses and increasing them as needed by small amounts. That would be better than missing insulin doses.

ROSA: Changing to a less expensive insulin helps me. I've really worried about missing my insulin.

PHYSICIAN: That's understandable. I am concerned about your stress and what you are doing with the insulin. The stress is serious. I'm also wondering whether you feel down or depressed also.

ROSA: I'm too busy for that. I feel full of pressure trying to keep my family going. I'm not sad, I feel more driven.

PHYSICIAN: What do you think would decrease the stress? (Evoking)

ROSA: I don't know.

PHYSICIAN: Would it be helpful to offer an idea for you to consider? (Asking permission before offering advice [E-P-E])

ROSA: Yes.

PHYSICIAN: You have an employee assistance plan at work that gives you three free visits to speak with a counselor. What do think about that idea?

ROSA: I feel a lot of pressure now. But I feel sort of embarrassed to talk about it.

PHYSICIAN: You have reservations about talking to someone. (Simple reflection) I have no intention of pushing something on you. Would it be OK to ask a question? (Asking permission and respecting autonomy)

ROSA: OK.

PHYSICIAN: Can you think of any benefits at all from speaking with a counselor?

ROSA: I'm pretty worried right now. I can see how talking with someone might help me. (Preparatory change talk) But I hate to miss work now because I lose income. (A mix of change talk followed by sustain talk)

PHYSICIAN: You feel like you would get some relief by speaking with someone. (Reflection focusing only on the preparatory change talk)

ROSA: Probably. Years ago I saw a counselor when I was in college. I was short of money then too. I worked my way through college.

PHYSICIAN: You felt better because the stress was relieved. (A complex reflection that makes a guess [that the stress was relieved])

ROSA: It helped me. I probably need to do that now. (Change talk)

PHYSICIAN: What would help you make the decision to do that? (Evoking that mobilizes change talk)

ROSA: I would have to ask for certain weekdays off so I'd be able to go.

PHYSICIAN: That's a way for you to do this. (Simple reflection)

ROSA: Yes.

Focusing and Evoking

This brief conversation was guided toward evoking. It began with the patient focusing on glycemic control and her A1c level. The physician avoided direct confrontation or judgments about her increased A1c level by evoking her thoughts about what caused it. This was followed by a brief screening for distress. Rosa volunteered details about her stressful situation.

In the next part of the conversation, the physician expanded focusing to include treatment for Rosa's diabetes and continued evoking until Rosa said "I don't know" when asked about what would relieve her distress. Using E-P-E in response to the patient's statement, "I don't know," provided an opportunity to discuss less expensive insulins for treating her diabetes.

The last part of the discussion focused on treating the primary cause of Rosa's significantly increased A1c level, psychological distress. In the course of this conversation there was a brief query about depression and that did not appear to be a notable concern. Evoking continued to play an important part, with Rosa using preparatory change talk. As occurred in this encounter, an open question ended up evoking Rosa's mobilizing change talk.

Using sedative medications for psychological distress in diabetes is not an ideal option. There is little evidence to support it, and it does not address the cause(s) of the stress. Mental health conditions that stand in the way of diabetes self-care are more comprehensively treated when diabetes professionals join with mental health professionals who can help their patients.

Depression Magnifies the Challenges of Diabetes

The literature on diabetes and depression is ponderous and chilling. Depression occurs in people with T1D and T2D at a rate more than twice that of people without diabetes (Anderson et al., 2001). The disruptions caused by this mood disorder result in impaired self-care and the onset or worsening of diabetic complications (Lin et al., 2004). Depression is easily missed because of the significant diabetes problems occurring as depression evolves. The diabetes problems necessitate attention. However, they can easily camouflage depression. Research has shown that depression is frequently missed or undertreated in people with diabetes and other chronic conditions (Chaoyang, Ford, Guixiang, Bakkuz, & Mokdad, 2010; Hudson et al., 2013; Li et al., 2010).

To improve outcomes, it is necessary to identify the people in your practice who have depression. Once they are identified, follow-up is essential to ensure that the person receives adequate treatment. Included in this chapter are examples of using MI in conversations about screening, treatment, or referral for treatment. Before focusing on ways of identifying people in your practice who have depression, let us present an overview of the problems associated with it, which should heighten the value of your knowing who has it.

Imagine the difficulties a person experiences when he first learns he has had long-standing diabetes when hospitalized for treatment of a first heart attack. Or consider the challenges of a person also experiencing a myocardial infarction after years of working hard to avoid diabetic complications. Diabetes causes problems that can lead to depression. In a meta-analysis of depression in diabetes, the percentage of people with depression was 31% (Anderson et al., 2001). In people without diabetes the percentage with depression was much lower, 14% (Anderson et al., 2001). This means that in the average diabetes practice, 3 out of 10 patients may have concomitant depression.

The results from depression can be severe for people with diabetes. In a group of 4,263 people with T2D followed for 5 years, those who developed MDD (major depressive disorder) or PDD (persistent depressive disorder, also known as dysthymia) had a significantly higher incidence of complications—blindness, end-stage renal disease, amputations (from inadequate circulation and/or diabetic sensory neuropathy that lead to diabetic ulcers that fail to heal), myocardial infarction, and stroke (Lin et al., 2010). The disengagement from activities associated with depression results in people skipping medications, blood glucose monitoring, annual eye exams, regular foot exams, and healthy eating (Lin et al., 2004).

Depression undermines work and family wellness, too. Partners of depressed people with T2D experience distress or depressive symptoms at levels as great as or greater than their partner (Fisher, Chesla, Skaff, Mullan, & Kanter, 2002). Depression is also linked to psychosomatic symptoms that increase health care encounters and absences from work (Druss, Rosenheck, & Sledge, 2000; Katon, 2009).

Partners of depressed people with T2D experience distress or depressive symptoms at levels as great as or greater than their partner.

Mental health resources were limited or completely absent in the rural and frontier locations where I have worked for most of my career. I have always enjoyed behavioral health. So, my continuing education time was often spent at programs on mental health topics, especially depression, other mood disorders, and training in pharmacotherapy. In the late 1990s and early 2000s, as the chronic care model was being widely discussed, I read, studied, and met with people to explore collaborative care models for rural settings. The results of that inquiry led to the inclusion of a part-time nurse and dietitian in our diabetes care program. Later we also hired a licensed professional counselor to work I day a week in our office. Our diabetes education program also became recognized by the American Diabetes Association. This work was supported robustly by the rural hospital and clinic where I worked. It was an exciting time. Our diabetes care benefited greatly from those decisions. I have great respect for the work done by the people we hired, some of whom drove well over a hundred miles through rural Montana in their commute to our clinic.

Later on, when I moved to a larger community, I initially lacked a group of people with whom to work. I started first by calling mental health professionals who often told me they would like to help my patients, but they knew very little about diabetes. My response caught them off guard: "I know very little about eating disorders or chemical dependency disorders" (depending on the profession of the person with whom I was speaking). The phone calls frequently led to meeting in a restaurant for a meal and discussing how we would work together. I enjoyably learned that there were nurses, nurse practitioners, dietitians, and mental health professionals who were willing to help me by providing consultations and care to the people I was seeing. I learned that collaborative care is not only a sponsored institution-based service. Taking the time to call and meet a colleague can create collaborative care.

—MPS

Perhaps the most impressive and disturbing aspects of MDD and PDD are on mortality. Lin et al. (2004) reported on a group of 4,184 people with diabetes. Over the course of almost 5 years, 428 people without depression died, 12.9% of the group. Among the group with MDD, 88 people (17.8%) died. Of those with PDD, 65 people (18.2%) died. For those with MDD and PDD, the hazard ratios for death (adjusted for demographic, clinical characteristics, health habits, and disease control level) were 1.52 and 1.24, respectively. The vast majority of the deaths were related to diabetic complications, overwhelming sepsis, cancer, and chronic obstructive pulmonary disease (Lin et al., 2009). The deaths from pulmonary disease may have occurred because, compared to people with diabetes alone, twice the number of people with diabetes and depression also smoke cigarettes (Lin et al., 2004).

A meta-analysis of 16 studies on depression and mortality risk concluded that depression increased the hazard ratio for people with diabetes and depression to 1.5 (van Dooren et al., 2013). Putting this into perspective, the hazard ratio for dying in people with diabetes alone is increased to 1.4, compared to the nondiabetic population (hazard ratio =1.0) (Williams et al., 2012). Increasing an already elevated mortality hazard ratio for diabetes means that, with both diabetes and depression, people double the risk of dying (hazard ratio = 2.13 for MDD and 1.96 for PDD).

Screening People for Depression

Amid all the negative outcomes for people with diabetes there is the good news that depression can be detected and adequately treated. Collaborative care, using case managers working with the patient, their diabetes care providers, specialists, and mental health professionals, has shown evidence for effective treatment. This team approach has been demonstrated to be effective in several studies. The Pathways Study compared the treatment of depression and diabetes in primary care practices. Two groups of patients with depression and two or more diabetes complications were compared to patients with two or less diabetic complications. Depression scores improved twofold in people with two or more diabetic complications who received collaborative care for MDD as compared to those receiving usual care (Kinder et al., 2006).

A meta-analysis of eight studies also showed that this team-based approach for MDD or PDD provided benefits to people with T2D. Compared to a usual care control group, the intervention group receiving collaborative care had significantly greater improvements of depression scores, a response ratio of 1.53. The response ratios for taking antidepressants and oral hypoglycemic medications also were higher, 1.79 and 2.18, respectively. There were no differences, however, in the A1c levels for people in the intervention groups or usual care groups (Huang, Wei, Wu, Chen, & Guo, 2013).

In a recent study nurse case managers coordinated care among primary care medical practices, a multidisciplinary group of consultants (including mental health professionals and pharmacists) and patients. The nurses worked to facilitate three areas of medication use—medications for diabetes, preventive care (statins and blood pressure medications), and depression. They also worked with patients to improve problem-solving skills and motivation. Working with physicians, they also helped patients make adjustments in medications for diabetes and depression.

The results were impressive. Collaborative care helped people improve control over their depression. It also increased their willingness to provide more effective diabetes self-care. Compared to those receiving usual care, the experimental group had adjustments for antidepressant medications six times more frequently. There were threefold higher adjustment rates for the use of insulin and almost twice as many more adjustment rates for antihypertensive and statin medications in the intervention group. Additionally, people in the intervention group more frequently self-monitored their blood glucose levels and blood pressure. Regular monitoring using the Patient Health Questionnaire–9 (PHQ-9) confirmed improvements in depression (Lin et al., 2012).

The high incidence of depression in diabetes along with the harmful experiences people have in health, family life, work, and overall quality of life justify regularly screening for depression. In their standards of care for diabetes, the American Diabetes Association (2014, pp. 532–533) recommends screening for mental health problems: "Routinely screen for psychosocial problems such as depression and diabetes-related distress, anxiety, eating disorders, and cognitive impairment."

The PHQ-9 effectively screens for MDD. It is widely used in medical practices and health care research (Kroenke, Spitzer, & Williams, 2001), performing well as a screening tool, with a sensitivity of 88% and a specificity of 88% for MDD (Kroenke et al., 2001).

The PHQ-9 is designed to be self-administered. It is based on the major and minor symptoms of MDD. Patients can complete it while waiting to be seen or during their appointment. In the single instructions page there is a helpful numeric assessment that measures depression severity. The scale has been used in research and could be used in your office to determine initially and over time the person's response to treatment. It is easy for practitioners to score the results, a feature that facilitates discussions of the results before the patient leaves the office. Adequately treating depression is important. When patients do not respond fully to treatment in a way that resolves their depression, chronic depression can create a long-term disability.

Screening programs are most helpful when all of the target population, people with diabetes, is screened regularly. A useful way to do this is to screen annually and episodically when you are seeing people with symptoms of MDD or deterioration in diabetes control. One way to approach screening for depression is to tell people in your practice that you are concerned about the risks of depression:

"Each year there are questions I ask all my patients about depression. It is something that can really impact your diabetes and overall health. Would it be all right to talk about that now?"

Obtaining permission and sharing with people that this is a routine discussion is important. It expresses your concern for them and decreases the stress and hesitancy that might otherwise occur if people felt singled out for a mental health condition.

The following interview is an example of screening when there is a clinical concern about a significant increase in A1c level. The conversation includes reflective listening, asking permission, affirmations, and eliciting the patient's ideas.

> PRACTITIONER: Since your last visit, your A1c has increased from 7.2% to 8.8%. What are your thoughts about that? (Evoking)
>
> PATIENT: I have a lot going on now. One of my kids is having problems in school. I didn't realize it until the teacher and principal told me last week that he has been having behavior problems at school for 2 months. I wish they had told me sooner.
>
> PRACTITIONER: You're dealing with a difficult new problem. (Simple reflection)
>
> PATIENT: It feels like a problem that can't be fixed. My husband doesn't seem concerned about it at all. We were already having problems getting along before the school contacted me.
>
> PRACTITIONER: It is not just your son; it's also your husband. And both of those problems are burdensome. How have you been feeling? (A complex reflection followed by an open question)
>
> PATIENT: I feel edgy, sort of anxious about things because I'm not sure what to do. I wake up real early in the morning thinking about all of this. Sometimes during the day when I'm by myself I feel so alone. We're having so many arguments at home.
>
> PRACTITIONER: When people with diabetes are stressed out or feeling down, their A1c levels often increase. I wonder what you know about depression. (Evoking)
>
> PATIENT: It involves feeling sad. I wondered about depression. But I've never been depressed before. I know that medicines and counselors are used to treat it.
>
> PRACTITIONER: You're right, that's how it's treated. And you have good insights about the situation you are in. (Affirmations) You probably remember the annual screening for depression that I do. You've participated in it before. I also encourage people to be rescreened during the year if they have some of the symptoms of depression. Would you be willing to complete this questionnaire now? (Asking permission)
>
> PATIENT: Yes.

Although the patient had obvious symptoms of depression, using the PHQ-9 is still helpful. The depression severity score before treatment can be used sequentially to monitor the adequacy of treatment.

The spirit and skills of MI are helpful in the sensitive area of depression screening. Many people have reservations and uneasiness about visiting mental health clinicians. Depression can heighten the anxiety and stress more. Uncontrolled diabetes with recurrent hypoglycemia and/or hyperglycemia can exacerbate depression, especially among people with chronic diabetic complications (Hedayati et al., 2009). This can become so severe that people with long-standing uncontrolled diabetes may elect to abandon efforts at self-care. Although it may not be mentioned, the patient likely has remorse about his or her inability to provide effective self-care. Downplaying self-care or detachment from apparent problems are ways of avoiding discussions of sensitive material.

MI is especially suited to working with people in the midst of such challenging circumstances. Compassion, accurate empathy, and evoking provide a safe environment to discuss sensitive topics. People feel understood.

There are other practical areas in which MI is useful. Some people are leery of having a mental health diagnosis and therefore minimize their symptoms and their need for treatment. MI is a viable way to work with people who feel this way.

The following interview features a physician assistant who is working with Dan, a patient who just completed the PHQ-9. It was not a part of the routine annual screening. It was done because Dan discontinued taking his statin and antihypertensive medications, and his A1c levels had risen from 7.2% to 8.8% since his last visit 3 months earlier. The dialogue unfolds following a statement from the physician assistant. He told Dan that the results of the screening indicate the likelihood of having moderately severe depression. Dan questions the results of the screening.

PHYSICIAN ASSISTANT: You don't feel the screening is correct. (A simple reflection based on what Dan said previously)

DAN: That's right. I've never had mental problems in the past.

PHYSICIAN ASSISTANT: You're concerned about the possibility of a mental health disorder. And it's hard for you to consider that. The feelings you have are strong. You don't feel comfortable with this possibility. (A complex reflection) Would it be all right if I asked you a question to help me understand this better? (Asking permission)

DAN: I guess so.

PHYSICIAN ASSISTANT: Can you tell me what you know about depression? (Evoking)

DAN: It means being sad. Mood is turned way down. That's not the way I feel. When you asked on the questionnaire if I was feeling sad, I told you I didn't feel that way very much.

PHYSICIAN ASSISTANT: That's right, you did tell me that. You also said that you have little interest or enjoyment in doing things almost every day. Many people with depression don't feel sad. Instead they don't enjoy their lives. They often stop engaging in activities they used to enjoy. What are your thoughts about what I've just said? (Reflections followed by evoking)

DAN: I never thought that not doing things or enjoying them was a big part of depression. I thought depression was more like sadness. Something's changed in me; I know that. But I don't want to take another medicine for a new problem. I'm already having problems taking all the medicines I'm supposed to take.

PHYSICIAN ASSISTANT: You're just starting to think that maybe there is something awry. And you don't want to take another medication to treat it. (Using reflections to agree with the patient) What do you know about the treatment of depression? (Evoking)

DAN: Well, not very much. And I'm not sure I have it, either. But I know that people take medicine for depression. And I guess some people talk with counselors about it. This is my first go-round with something like this, and I don't know much about it.

PHYSICIAN ASSISTANT: You're accurate about treatment. Most of the treatment for it is speaking with a therapist and/or using medication. One thing for sure, though, you don't like how you feel right now. (Complex reflection)

DAN: You're right on the last thing you said. I have concerns, even if I'm not doing much.

PHYSICIAN ASSISTANT: I'm thinking from what you've said that you want to be sure that it is depression. Maybe then it would be easier to decide what to do about it. (A guess added to the reflection)

DAN: Yes, and I'm saying that only because I know what I don't want but I'm not sure about what I do want.

PHYSICIAN ASSISTANT: You don't feel sure you have depression. Would it be helpful if I provided some advice and information? (Asking permission)

DAN: OK.

PHYSICIAN ASSISTANT: I'm wondering if it would be helpful to consult with a psychologist or a counselor who could discuss this with you and offer an opinion. Depression is treatable. A second opinion about this might be helpful. Psychologists and counselors have a lot of experience treating depression. What are your thoughts about what I've said?

DAN: Look, what I'm having trouble with is having a mental condition.

Finding out I did might not be helpful. I've got trouble already getting done with all the things I have to do right now.

PHYSICIAN ASSISTANT: You told me earlier you are having problems getting things done. You also seem to be struggling with the idea that the reason you can't get things done is because you're depressed.

DAN: Exactly.

PHYSICIAN ASSISTANT: I wonder what the risks are of not getting the things done that are important to you. (An open question)

DAN: The things I have to do now just don't seem important to me. But they matter to my family and my boss at work. It is a busy time for me at work right now.

PHYSICIAN ASSISTANT: Your family is important to you. You want things to go well for them. And work is demanding. You want to do a good job. The way you feel makes you worried about getting important things done.

DAN: Umm . . . I would hate to miss a day at work now. It would make me feel like I failed. I've sort of done that with my diabetes already.

PHYSICIAN ASSISTANT: You don't want to miss work or lose your job. I know you don't like the idea of seeing a psychologist. There is no way I could make you do that, either. The choice is yours. But do you think there could be any potential benefits or advantages to seeing a psychologist?

DAN: I don't know. I do know that I can't afford to get in trouble at work or get sick from not taking care of my diabetes.

PHYSICIAN ASSISTANT: You don't want to lose your job or have complications from your health. It would really bother you if that happened. What do you think you should do?

DAN: Do you think I could make just one visit to see what it's like?

PHYSICIAN ASSISTANT: Sure. I can give you some names and you could call them. How would that work for you?

DAN: I should call somebody before my problems at work get worse.

PHYSICIAN ASSISTANT: I understand . . . that makes sense. Sometimes when people get stressed or depressed, they begin to have thoughts about hurting themselves or committing suicide. Is that something you've been experiencing?

DAN: I have thought about suicide a time or two.

PHYSICIAN ASSISTANT: Have you thought about or planned how you would do it?

DAN: No! My family is too important to me. I love them.

PHYSICIAN ASSISTANT: It would be good for us to get together after you see the psychologist. If it's all right with you, our nurse will call you to be sure you were able to make the appointment.

DAN: That's OK. It is hard to get appointments with some people.

PHYSICIAN ASSISTANT: She could help you with that if you have problems getting an appointment.

DAN: Thanks.

Caveats in Depression Care

An important area related to depression is suicide prevention. As in the interview above, suicide questions focus on two areas: first, "Do you think of committing suicide?" and, second, "Do you have a plan for doing so?" If a person affirmatively answers the second question, he should be referred for an emergency mental health consultation for assessment of suicidal risk. It is not uncommon for depressed people to say they have thought about suicide. If a person is thinking of suicide and the thoughts seem compelling or constant, even in the absence of a specific suicide plan, mental health consultation should be provided on an urgent basis.

Most people with depression do not have suicide plans, but follow-up is an essential part of working with people who have MDD or PDD. Whether you are providing diabetes care only or care for diabetes and depression, patients initially need additional regular care for both until they are stabilized. Collaborative care is helpful. Phone calls from a nurse ideally with case management and MI experience can facilitate self-care in diabetes and depression, especially if the nurse has a way to easily confer with treating practitioners.

Key Points

- Ask patients annually or more often if you have suspicions they are experiencing the symptoms of psychological distress, such as anxiety, stress, and/or worries. The symptoms can be related to diabetes or nondiabetes areas of life. In either area, the effect is cumulative.

- Sedative medications are not a good choice for diabetes-related stress. Look for the root causes (as was done in the interview above) and consider mental health referrals.

- When self-care appears compromised, think of obstacles that complicate diabetes—substance use, psychological distress, or depression. If these obstacles are not treated, diabetes-based recommendations alone are likely to go unheeded.

- Depression occurs twice as frequently among people with diabetes. Symptoms of depression can be subtle and easy to overlook because of the serious diabetic problems caused by depression.

- MI fits well into discussions that explore sensitive topics such as depression.

- The PHQ-9 is a good way to screen for depression. Its depression severity scale provides a helpful way to assess the effectiveness of treatment. Those not responding should be referred expeditiously to mental health professionals.

- Treatment for depression in diabetes is a team activity. Collaborative care greatly improves outcomes.

CHAPTER 14

Talking with the Family

amily members accompany people with T2D to all sorts of diabetes-related appointments, and most of the time visits in the presence of a family member go smoothly. For example, a potentially positive influence is present when dietitians see patients for medical nutrition therapy. If the person purchasing groceries and cooking the meals is present, this can facilitate healthier eating for a family member who has diabetes. However, the roles of spouses or partners, adult family members, and grandchildren, and even of friends or neighbors who accompany someone to a diabetes appointment, can also create ambiguity for clinicians, who wonder about their roles.

The following exchange occurs when Cheryl, a 56-year-old woman diagnosed with T2D 1 month earlier, returns to her dietitian's office for another appointment. The dietitian has not yet met Cheryl's husband, Frank, who accompanies her to this appointment. She has lost weight since her last visit—her body mass index (BMI) has dropped from 31.7 to 31.2 kg/m^2. Her A1c level has also dropped from 9.7% (when she was first diagnosed) to 8.4% today. Cheryl has a long history of obesity and sensitivity to criticism.

DIETITIAN: (*smiling warmly at Cheryl and her husband*) Cheryl, it's nice to see you today. You must be Frank. Our office assistant told me you came in with your wife today. (*They shake hands.*)

CHERYL: My husband never stops giving me advice; he's always telling me what I need to do. So, I thought it might be good for him to join us today.

FRANK: I'm concerned about you . . . losing weight would help your diabetes.

CHERYL: I know that. I'm working on it.

DIETITIAN: Frank, you care about your wife and want to help her. How's that been going for each of you? (Evoking with a complex reflection, followed by an open question)

CHERYL: Frank wants me to be successful with my diabetes, but I'm the one who needs to figure out all of this stuff. I can do that on my own. I'm the one who has to take care of it.

FRANK: (*smiling*) I have a difficult job. She told me she needed to give up big breakfasts, but she's still eating a lot of greasy food for breakfast. You really haven't taken care of that, have you?

In this brief conversation, the contentiousness is palpable. A family member who volunteers to be the diabetes "police officer" often stimulates arguments and may even have the paradoxical effect of eliciting pushback. This sort of contentious behavior relates to the findings from an interesting study of African American families that included a member with T2D. The study created four focus groups recruited from adult volunteers with and without T2D. Each volunteer was either living in a household with someone who had T2D or the person volunteering had T2D. The study design did not necessarily include family members related to one another in each group. The authors identified various types of well-intentioned communications of information or advice that actually compromised communication in the focus groups and in their families. As the authors examined the dysfunction in diabetes-related conversations, they observed that both the people with T2D and family members without T2D found it so difficult to communicate that many of them gave up attempting to be understood by one another, resulting in what the authors described as a "diabetes silence" (Samuel-Hodge, Cene, Corsino, Thomas, & Svetkey, 2013).

Silence, the antithesis of communication, unfortunately cuts off a potentially supportive relationship; it leaves the person with diabetes unable to share important discussions about the bothersome or successful aspects of his/her diabetes self-care. Although the study focused on African American families similar issues occur in other groups of people with diabetes. The righting reflex (See Chapter 1) is not just something within the aegis of health care practitioners. Many people faced with concerns about a loved one, a close friend, or even a work associate want the best outcomes for the person. The desired intention to help can actually overturn helpfulness. Like Cheryl, people are compelled in many instances to make their *own* conundrums workable. Even when people are struggling with a sizable challenge, the only reliable signals of a need for help is a request for it or a willingness to receive it, once the health care professional has asked permission to provide it.

There is a growing body of evidence that suggests that the troublesome impact of T2D does not only affect the individual who has it. Rather, the spouses of people who have T2D and/or depression or anxiety also develop significant symptoms of depression or anxiety, at times worse than those of the person with diabetes (Fisher et al., 2002).

Many of the people who accompany patients to your office for T2D care are spouses. Although marital relationships offer significant benefits, problems sometimes occur. This was the focus of a 2010 meta-analysis looking at the impact of couple-oriented interventions on chronic conditions. It examined the health of people with chronic conditions and the negative aspects of the condition on the spouses. Twenty-five studies were selected across a range of chronic conditions, such as cancer, chronic pain, arthritis, HIV infection, and T2D. The goal was to identify care interventions that were beneficial to both parties. The meta-analysis concluded that there were too few studies comparing patient-centered and couple-centered interventions to improve outcomes. However, the researchers did add that couple-centered approaches to improving care had small positive effects on the patient. These effects decreased the symptoms of patients with depression, improved marital functioning, and ameliorated pain, suggesting that couple-based interventions might work better for couples with illness-related discord, limited partner support, and lower-quality marital relationships (Martire, Schulz, Helgeson, Small, & Saghafi, 2010).

Despite the fact that people with diabetes are frequently accompanied to their appointments by another person, research on this outpatient phenomenon is scarce. In 2011, an interesting study focused on the participation of family members or friends (called companions in the study) during primary care visits with patients who had diabetes or congestive heart failure. This study appeared to be one of the first of its kind. The authors surveyed 439 patients with those conditions and 88 primary care physicians. The patients' ages ranged from 25 to 95, with 41% of them between 51 and 64 years old. Fifty-four percent of respondents were men, and 68% of the patients were married. The average length of the physician–patient relationships was 6.9 years.

Friends or family members attended almost half (48%) of the scheduled appointments. Forty-four percent of the patients reported it was easier for them to discuss difficult topics when their companions were present, and 77% stated that they had a better understanding of the physician's advice. Almost all the physicians, 95%, reported that when companions were present they had a better understanding of the patients' concerns. The doctors also stated that 71% of the companions contradicted information the patient had provided. However, physicians reported that in only 18% of the visits did the companions provide information that the patients did not want them to provide. In 6–7% of the visits, there was conflict

> *Almost all the physicians, 95%, reported that when companions were present they had a better understanding of the patients' concerns.*

between the patient and the companion. Importantly patients whose visits regularly occurred with their companion were more likely to report high satisfaction with the visits (Rosland, Piette, Choi, & Heisler, 2011).

Communication in Families

Before returning to Cheryl and Frank, it is helpful to consider communication in families. People with diabetes have much to gain from supportive, compassionate family members. However, if the gain ends up placing sizable burdens on the helper, the capacity of someone to assist on a long-term basis can be injured. The demands of continuous daily care for diabetes can easily cause both helpers and people with diabetes to burn out.

The brief exchange in the opening dialogue was telling. Cheryl wants to develop her own approach for the self-care tasks confronting her. With newly diagnosed diabetes, people need time to safely experiment with self-care to learn what will work for them. Frank, however, is dismayed by his wife's consumption of high fat content breakfasts and her obesity. His suggestions in those areas have become irritating to Cheryl. Discord, rather than collaborative support, makes diabetes self-care even more difficult for Cheryl. Even though she has done well in the first month of diagnosed T2D, she is not completely satisfied. So, she decided to invite Frank to join her, maybe hoping the clinician will become the referee she is looking for to end their disputes.

The way they communicate raises concerns about how well Frank understands his spouse's needs. Is this a patterned way of communicating developed over time dealing with previous stressful situations they have confronted? Long-standing patterns of unhelpful communication are more likely to get sorted out and better addressed in family therapy than in a diabetes care setting. Facing the difficulties of a chronic disorder and the potential for serious complications is easier in a climate of support. Exploring the couple's willingness to focus on how they are communicating in the office can help you understand better whether they are ready and willing to discuss Cheryl's new diagnosis and how they are communicating about it. It also offers an important clue as to whether this is a long-standing pattern in discussions about stressful topics or instead an atypical response caused by the acute stress from Cheryl's recent diagnosis of diabetes. As you will soon see, the dietitian did not pursue examining their communication styles because the focus of the visit did not allow for it.

As we return to Cheryl and Frank, you can see that working with them could be challenging: the jab about unhealthy breakfasts that Frank delivered after Cheryl's attempt to declare ownership of her diabetes self-care could cause some practitioners to take sides with one or the other of them.

CHERYL: I'm not going to continue the arguments we have at home when I'm here, Frank. Can you understand that, Frank?

FRANK: (*Looks down silently.*)

DIETITIAN: You've done a good job losing weight since your last visit, 22 pounds—and also your average blood glucose has dropped from 230 to 193[mg/dl].

CHERYL: I know I've lost weight. I've cut out sweet things like sodas completely.

DIETITIAN: That's hard work, a great accomplishment for you! So, what would you like to focus on today? (An affirmation followed by an open question)

CHERYL: Even though I was able to stop drinking sodas, I still like to eat too much. When I cut down on the sweet sodas, I started drinking lots of diet soda instead. I'm eating more fatty food because it does not make my blood glucose go as high. Frank's right about that.

DIETITIAN: You have positive and negative feelings about what's going on. You feel good about the big change you made in soda sweetened with sugar and you're concerned because you can't curb your attraction to food. (Complex reflection that makes a guess)

FRANK: That's what you've said at home, Cheryl.

CHERYL: It makes me feel good when I'm eating. It's been that way for most of my life. I've been overweight since I was a child. [Focuses on her attraction to food rather than her recent successes.]

DIETITIAN: You have a lot of concern about this. You've thought about this for a long time.

CHERYL: I haven't stopped thinking about it for years, long before I got diabetes.

DIETITIAN: Do you have any ideas about what would help you deal with this? (Evoking her solution to the problem)

CHERYL: I don't know . . . it bothers me a lot, and not just because of Frank's constant reminders.

FRANK: It bothers me too.

CHERYL: I know it does, but you're just as overweight as I am . . . you don't have much room to talk to me about it.

FRANK: But I don't have diabetes.

DIETITIAN: Cheryl, you're worried about your attraction to food, and that's something that's concerned you for a long time. (A reiteration of the dietitian's previous complex reflection) You want to do something about it. (A reiteration of the reflection that makes a guess)

CHERYL: I just don't know. Yeah . . . I'm concerned. But I don't want to fail, and I think I probably would fail if I tried to do something about this problem.

DIETITIAN: Would it be OK for me to ask about a sensitive topic? You don't have to make a response if you don't want to talk about it. (Asking permission and respecting autonomy)

CHERYL: You can ask the question, but you're right. I might not want to talk about it.

DIETITIAN: What do you know about eating disorders?

CHERYL: There's a lot of stuff in that question. I know I use food when I'm feeling stressed out. That goes way back.

DIETITIAN: That's right. Eating disorders can involve the use of food as a way of calming down when you're stressed out. (An affirmation of Cheryl's insight)

CHERYL: I actually know a lot about eating disorders, and I'll tell you right now I don't want to go back to that guy in town who advertises that he knows how to treat people with eating problems. I've already tried him out.

FRANK: I'm willing to go with you again if that would help.

CHERYL: You'd go with me? You've got to be joking! You need to see somebody like that as much as I do. We're both overweight, Frank. You may not have diabetes, but you can't control your eating either.

DIETITIAN: There are several people in town that treat eating disorders. How would it work if I gave you the names of therapists other than the one you saw in the past? (An open question)

CHERYL: I don't want to fail at something this important.

DIETITIAN: Can you help me understand what you mean by failure?

CHERYL: I'd sneak around eating secretly. And I hate to do that.

DIETITIAN: Can I offer some information about what you said? (Asking permission)

CHERYL: All right.

DIETITIAN: When people work on changing a difficult area in their life, the change doesn't turn on like a light switch. They go back and forth between where they were and over time move closer to where they want to be. What are your thoughts about that? (Information followed by evoking Cheryl's input)

CHERYL: I've been through this stuff before. I know that.

DIETITIAN: When you came in today, this was the topic you wanted to discuss. I'm wondering if you can think of any benefit at all to seeing a therapist to talk about your eating habits.

CHERYL: Talking with someone might help me deal with him. (*Points her finger at Frank.*) (Change talk)

FRANK: Now you're the one who's got to be joking. I'm trying to help you!

CHERYL: Almost always you give me a hard time about what I might not be able to do.

DIETITIAN: There are two issues in front of us now. (A simple reflection)

CHERYL: What do you mean?

DIETITIAN: You're concerned about Frank's criticism, something you find quite irritating and you also think it's important to do something about the way you eat. (A compound and complex reflection)

An uncomfortable silence lasting almost 2 minutes begins.

CHERYL: The two problems you're referring to are not easy for me to deal with because I've been struggling with them for most of my life. These things go way back.

DIETITIAN: And even though they are long-standing and difficult for you to live with, overeating was what you said was important to discuss at your visit today. What are the benefits to you of not doing something about this?

CHERYL: I feel I can't live down failure if I continue my way of eating after trying again. I've tried a lot in the past. I couldn't even succeed when I knew I might get diabetes. Look, this isn't just about food.

DIETITIAN: This topic is painful for you. (Empathy) Your willingness to bring it up today, after weight loss and improvement in A1c indicates you want to do well. (Affirmation) I can help you with care for your diabetes. I'm not qualified to help you with your eating addiction. (Provides information that ethically pertains to this situation) I'm also concerned that the overeating makes your diabetes self-care more difficult. I can't force you to do something about it. (Respecting autonomy)

CHERYL: I have to think about this. I do need to do something, and I have to really concentrate on how to go about doing this. (Commitment to consider change)

DIETITIAN: That's a wonderful idea. (Affirmation) I am available if you want to discuss this after thinking about it.

CHERYL: I'm grateful for your willingness to see me. If I figure something out, I would like to speak with you about it before I make an appointment with someone else. I'm going to work on this. I appreciate your putting up with us today.

FRANK: That's the truth.

DIETITIAN: So, today we spoke about your recent success with weight loss and the improvements in your blood glucose values. You are concerned that you eat more when you're stressed out. You want to think seriously about seeing a new, different therapist for help with your patterns of overeating when stressed and to help find a way to deal with the criticism you receive. We can help you with getting an appointment if you decide to do so. Does that sound correct? (Reflective summary)

CHERYL: Yes, it does. Should I come back to see you?

DIETITIAN: Yes, in about 1 month.

CHERYL: I'll do that.

Ambivalence, Discord and Silence

It appears as though Cheryl has locked herself in a prison of ambivalence. She is filled with the fear of not being able to overcome her food addiction and not being able to deal with a husband who relies on criticizing her. Yet she uses preparatory change talk about her *desire* to explore change and her *need* to do something about the problems. In the interview, she even makes a commitment to thinking about how she could tackle this momentous change. Ambivalence is a normal part of life; people experience it regularly in the course of their lives. In health care the resolution of ambivalence is necessary before embarking on change, especially when the change is as difficult as it is in Cheryl's case. The value of using MI to help people resolve ambivalence is widely recognized in a variety of situations.

So if ambivalence can be resolved, why do some people linger in it for long periods of time, even after visits with competent practitioners using MI? When ambivalence is entrenched and does not resolve with treatment, it is time to think of other obstacles co-occurring with it. Substance use disorders (treated in Chapter 12) are common, and—yes—food addiction is a good example of how dependency on food can obstruct the self-care of diabetes. The interviewer could have screened Cheryl for depression, but missed a good opportunity to do so. Living with someone like Frank raises the suspicion that this is a low-quality marital relationship. Combined with

Years ago I attended my first MI training led by a person who became a close friend and colleague, Chris Fiore. I moved to Missoula 1 year after the training, and we undertook regular meetings with another colleague, Steve Zellmer, to discuss MI and the challenging clinical opportunities we had to use it in our practices. I often think of something I learned toward the end of the first or second day of that first training. Chris brought up the topic of silence—those times when we are discussing something with people who are engaged and focused on the topic of discussion and then suddenly, after the clinician makes a statement, there is a period of silence (similar to what happened in the visit with Cheryl). The patient seems to just sit there. In my pre-MI days, I would quickly make a comment intended to propel the conversation forward. I was not comfortable with silence in clinical settings. Fortunately, I learned a different approach from Chris, one that I think has been more helpful for my patients and me. I just sit there and wait . . . for the silence to be broken. In fact I named it a pregnant silence. Pregnancy in the millennia before ultrasound left a couple wondering for nine months whether a girl or boy would be born. Metaphorically I wait in the same way, wondering: What idea will the patient deliver for both of us to explore? Silence has a discomfort associated with it. That discomfort can also become a creative tension. If we as practitioners resist the temptation to rescue people from that discomfort, we have time to wonder for an incredible, silent minute or two of the clinical dance as the person thinks, then says something, and the dance resumes anew.

—MPS

the trials of newly diagnosed diabetes, a burden of depression could fill to overflowing the backpack anyone uses to haul around the new routines of diabetes self-care. Marital problems, especially when they lead to depression, can also negatively affects one's capacity to meet challenges in other areas of life (Martire et al., 2010).

In a clinical setting like Cheryl's, a mental health consultation can potentially facilitate significant improvements in her quality of life. Does she need treatment or assessment for depression, an eating disorder, or family therapy with a difficult spouse? The answer is, "Yes." Any one of those situations is an indication for a mental health consultation. In the presence of all three of them, Cheryl's diabetes self-care and her health will be compromised until these co-occurring problems are effectively addressed.

The discord between Cheryl and Frank brings up an important topic in MI. Arguments or discord with patients are to be avoided. It always takes at least two people for discord to occur, and the responsibility for avoiding it belongs to the practitioner. The dietitian skillfully overlooked Frank's critical attitude and kept the mutual focus of the visit

It always takes at least two people for discord to occur, and the responsibility for avoiding it belongs to the practitioner.

clearly on Cheryl. There were only two mentions of Cheryl's difficulties with her husband—when the dietitian commented to her in passing about Frank's criticism and in her reflective summary.

Discord can also be triggered by staunch sustain talk (Miller & Rollnick, 2013, pp. 195–200). One might easily tire of listening to Cheryl's insecurities about her inability to work on her eating addiction. The dietitian instead helped Cheryl engage in the visit and did not attempt to resolve issues that were clearly under the aegis of mental health professionals. Instead, using E-P-E, the dietitian brought up the topic of mental health consultation and at the end of the conversation left it for Cheryl to consider. Fortunately, Cheryl chose to pick it up to ponder on her own. However, the value of mental health care was explored and the patient made a commitment to consider mental health consultation.

The difficulties posed during this encounter are often seen in diabetes care, even if people in your practice are not as contentious as Frank was. The consequences of eating disorders, substance use, depression, or stress are often long-standing when people are diagnosed with pernicious diabetic complications. MI offers a way to evoke from patients their plans and the steps they will take—hopefully, early in the course of diabetes—so that diabetic complications can be prevented or later ameliorated. Cheryl took the first steps down that path, thinking and considering about something very difficult for her to do, something she could seek additional support for in a follow-up visit, and something she could change.

Key Points

- When family members accompany a person with diabetes to his or her appointment there is an opportunity to view the effectiveness of their communication and how they support one another in challenging situations.

- MI skills and spirit can help you avoid discord with patients.

- MI helps people resolve ambivalence. If ambivalence does not get resolved, there may be other conditions that create obstacles to better health, including eating disorders, depression, and/or chronic psychological stress or substance use.

CHAPTER 15

Adolescents and Diabetes Self-Care

Most diabetes practitioners working with parents and their adolescent(s) with T1D find it challenging to help teenagers maintain glycemic control. Adolescence, defined by the American Academy of Pediatrics (2014) as the decade from 11 to 21 years of age, is associated with risky behavioral experiments. Although some people contend that experimentation can lead to better decision making in adulthood, T1D is a dangerous playing field for such experiments. For families, dangerous experiments with T1D contrast sharply with the longing that parents have for the safety and health of their teenager(s).

The health benefits of glycemic control for teenagers are significant. Complications in T1D develop based on both the length of time one has diabetes and the magnitude of uncontrolled hyperglycemia. The likelihood of diabetes-related complications is already greater for children and adolescents because they potentially have many more years of life with diabetes than people diagnosed later in life.

Adolescents differ from adult patients. The most important and obvious differences being their residence with and reliance on their parent(s) for support. It is important in diabetes care to have both the parent(s) and teenager participate in appointments together. Parents have significant responsibilities for their children, and their supportive involvement in diabetes self-care enhances their adolescent's self-efficacy (King, Berg, Butner, Butler, & Wiebe, 2014).

Whether adolescents with T1D come in on their own or in the company of their parents, the patient is not just the adolescent: the *family* is the patient. T1D in pediatric patients is a family activity—a team sport, not an individual one.

Adolescents need increased daily doses of insulin because they are rapidly growing, a process that creates insulin resistance. Teenagers often skip insulin doses, leading to significant hyperglycemia that can be long-lasting. Complications can and do occur during adolescence. In a prospective study of 94 children recruited between birth and 14 years of age and followed for an average of 12 years, 48% of them developed nonproliferative retinopathy (see Chapter 16) (Svensson, Eriksson, & Dahlquist, 2004). The study confirmed that higher A1c values, especially during the first 5 years of diabetes, predicted retinopathy. All children and adolescents deserve to have healthy, long lives as adults, but years of uncontrolled diabetes can diminish their chances of doing so.

Parents whose children have T1D assume much more complex responsibilities and tasks than the parents of children without diabetes. Self-care for T1D necessitates attention throughout the day and night. The work of diabetes self-care is so challenging that parents often develop stress when this emotionally laden work is imposed on already tightly scheduled days. The mother more often is the one most involved with the adolescent's diabetes self-care (Malerbi, Negrato, & Gomes, 2012). Sources of stress for the parents are related to worrying about hypoglycemia, hyperglycemia, and the risks for chronic complications from diabetes (Whittemore, Jaser, Chao, Jang, & Grey, 2012).

The tasks for parents are enormous. Depending on the ages of their offspring, parents perform, supervise, or verify the following diabetes-related tasks every day:

- Measuring of blood glucose values a minimum of four times daily
- Maintaining vigilance to detect the signs of hypoglycemia (young children are unable to recognize and treat hypoglycemia) or hyperglycemia
- Managing multiple insulin injections each day or the operation of an insulin pump
- Measuring or estimating the serving size for each meal or snack
- Carefully counting carbohydrate grams from food labels, personal lists, or memory
- Administering an accurate dose of insulin for the amount of food consumed
- Assuring that schools are providing appropriate support for both the education of their child and the school-based care needed by children with diabetes

The parents of adolescents with better glycemic control are generally mothers with higher levels of education (Haugstvedt, Wentzel-Larsen, Rokne, & Graue, 2011) and fathers with more authoritative (not authoritarian) parenting styles (Shorer et al., 2011). They are more likely to be in a higher socioeconomic group (Rosilio et al., 1998) and married (Urbach et al., 2005). A large multinational study also found that teenagers with better glycemic control rated their quality of life better than their peers with inadequate control (Hoey et al., 2001).

This good news is tempered by results from other studies. The T1D Exchange Clinic Network in the United States reported on a group of 7,203 teenagers (ages 13 to < 20 years old) with diabetes for more than 1 year. Most of the teens, 79%, had uncontrolled diabetes, based on an A1c level, ≥ 7.5% (Wood et al., 2013).

> *Most of the teens, 79%, had uncontrolled diabetes, based on an A1c level, ≥ 7.5%.*

Identifying specific targets for behavior change is an essential part of MI use. It is easy to identify behavioral targets in adolescents with uncontrolled diabetes, such as regular blood glucose testing, which is often minimized or discontinued by teenagers, resulting in uncontrolled hyperglycemia (Miller et al., 2013).

Blood glucose testing is not just a tool for satisfying the curiosity about one's current glucose level. Regular testing prompts behavioral self-care decisions, and in turn those decisions can lead toward improved diabetes outcomes. For example, in T1D the values are used to dose insulin needed to correct a high blood glucose level or to calculate how much insulin is needed to cover the carbohydrates in a meal or a snack and to verify whether or not hypoglycemia is present. Although many teenagers with uncontrolled diabetes say that they want a better A1c, regularly skipping self-monitored blood glucose testing distances them from that goal.

Mental health disorders in children and adolescents with T1D occur frequently. A recent study in Sweden enrolled 17,122 children with T1D and 18,847 of their healthy siblings between 1973 and 2009. They were followed until they were 18 years old. The risk of psychiatric problems in their first 6 months of diabetes was three-fold that of children without diabetes. Suicide attempts were increased 1.7 times in comparison to their peers without diabetes. After the 6-month interval psychiatric disorders were present in the children with diabetes twice as frequently as in children without diabetes. Their siblings without diabetes did not have an increased rate of psychiatric diagnoses. The study concluded that the etiology of mental health disorders in the children with diabetes was the result of having diabetes and not related to a genetic etiology (Butwicka, Frisen, Almqvist, Zethelius, & Lichtenstein, 2015).

Be aware of the potential need for mental health care when you are working with adolescents with diabetes and their families. The increased risks of mental health disorders along with the higher risks for diabetic complications justify this. Mental health care is essential for many families with adolescents who are struggling to improve diabetes control after multiple visits to diabetes professionals. The same recommendation applies to adolescents with the comorbidity of a mental health disorder, especially those recently diagnosed with diabetes (Butwicka et al., 2015). As demonstrated in the following interview, MI fits well in conversations focused on the need for mental health referrals.

Fifteen-year-old Jim, the teenager in the interview, has T1D of 5 years' duration. He lives with his mother Ann and two younger sisters in a single-parent family. They moved from a town 500 miles away 6 months earlier, just before Jim started 10th grade. He has only a few friends and has been bullied at school. This was discussed at his last doctor's appointment. He and his mother are also seeing a case manager who works for the local mental health agency and is able to maintain involvement with high-risk families. The physician also asked the case manager to facilitate an appointment with a family therapist because of the family's circumstances after mentioning to Ann that Jim probably has depression. Jim's A1c levels over the last year have gone up from 8.4%, before the move, to 10.5% following the move. His mother works full-time and does not get home from work until 6:00 P.M. The following interview is excerpted from their appointment after engaging with the case manager.

CASE MANAGER: Are there specific concerns that either of you have today? (Using an open question as focusing begins)

JIM: No.

ANN: He's not measuring his blood glucose very often, and he skips insulin at school and at home because I have to go to work early before school starts. I work a lot. I hate to say this, but I feel like I don't have enough time in my day to get everything done that needs to be done. I get stressed out by work and by Jim. I'm concerned about him because his A1c has gone up a lot. And I can't get him to take care of his diabetes. The kids that have been bullying him may have caused a lot of this.

CASE MANAGER: You are quite concerned about him being bullied. That's understandable. You want Jim's diabetes to be better controlled and are wondering if it would get better if the bullying stopped. What do you think should be done? (Evoking)

ANN: His doctor thought Jim was depressed. The doctor's like me—he can't get Jim to take better care of his diabetes. He said if he's depressed it could make it more difficult for him to take care of diabetes. If those kids stopped picking on him and he got treated for depression he might get better.

CASE MANAGER: You're right about his lack of treatment and the bullying. They could both be reasons for Jim's depression. (Affirming

Ann's insight) The case manager looks toward Jim. Jim, what do you know about depression? (Evoking)

JIM: Not much. People feel down when they're depressed. What bothers me is the work at school being a lot harder than it was at the school I was in last year.

CASE MANAGER: You're right about depression: people often feel down with it. (Affirmation) The fact that school is difficult really concerns you. School is even more difficult when other students are unfairly picking on you. (Complex reflection)

JIM: Yeah. And I don't have as many friends as I used to.

ANN: What do you expect? It took 3 years for you to make all those friends before we moved. We've just been here a few months.

CASE MANAGER: Things have been tough for you, Jim. And Ann, you're feeling challenged by all the work you have now. (Complex reflections) What did the doctor say about a referral to a family therapist? (The question expands focusing.)

ANN: He said it could be helpful for both of us. It's hard for me to get off work. I work at a grocery store. But I want to help my son. I talked to the people where I work today. They know Jim has diabetes, and I told them I might need to go to an appointment every week. They said they'd help me rearrange my work schedule. I hope I won't lose money doing it.

CASE MANAGER: I can really understand how difficult all this is for you and Jim. It's challenging to do things that could end up taking away some of your income. (Complex reflections) Would it be OK if I spoke with you about some ideas I have? (Seeking permission before providing information)

ANN: Sure, that's OK.

CASE MANAGER: I'm concerned about Jim's school and the difficulties he's having there. If you signed a consent for me to go to the school, I could speak with them about getting more help from the school nurse for his diabetes and investigate whether or not they know he's being bullied. He also may be eligible for other special services. What do each of you think about that? (E-P-E—asking for their thoughts/ideas after providing information)

JIM: I feel out of place there. If you go there, I hope things won't get worse for me.

CASE MANAGER: I can understand how you feel, Jim. I can assure that I would be talking to the staff. None of your classmates would know I even went there. The school has an obligation to make sure you are safe and not being picked on by other kids. I can speak with them about that.

JIM: I'd like it if those guys quit doing all that stuff.

ANN: Both of us need to see something good happening with that.

CASE MANAGER: I can understand Ann how difficult this is. (Empathy) If you are losing work and income from the appointments, let me know. I'm going to check to see if there is any way we could do something about that.

ANN: Well, that would be good. I'll talk to the school in the morning to let them know about you. I'll sign that form too.

CASE MANAGER: One other area is the family therapist. (Returns to focusing) What do you think about it?

ANN: He needs it. I'm so stressed and I hope it will help me, too.

CASE MANAGER: What do you think of going to family therapy Jim? (Evoking with an open question)

JIM: I'll go too.

All the health-related challenges families face in caring for T1D impact the quality of life and mental health of both parents and teenagers. This has clinical implications for MI use. Engaging parents and a teenager can be challenging, especially if there is discord in the family. The ways family members communicate with one another about improving diabetes self-care is an essential area to explore. There were difficulties for the family in the preceding interview.

Two questions can help you evaluate this area. First, can the parent(s) and adolescent(s) communicate effectively with one another? The brusque way Ann spoke to Jim when he mentioned his lack of friends raises concern. However, this concern is offset by her willingness to participate in family therapy and her worries about the conflicts at school. She also acknowledges she is under a lot of stress. If Jim's mother's communication is compromised at home in both diabetes and nondiabetes topics, their capacity to work together could be strained. Communicating effectively with a teenager who is aloof toward needed diabetes self-care is challenging enough.

It may be helpful to think of the righting reflex in the context of Jim's mother's remark. She wants to help him during this difficult set of circumstances, so she readily offers advice that may not be helpful in his current situation. Her comment about how long it takes to make friends is well intentioned but not expedient. It could intensify Jim's feelings of being overwhelmed by school, bullies, and the acute loss of the comforts associated with friends and routines he developed at their former residence.

The second question is whether family functioning is being altered by mental health issues that could stifle diabetes self-care and family functioning. Mental health disorders in parents and/or adolescents and poverty or minority status create barriers that hamper self-care (Cameron, Northam, Ambler, & Daneman, 2007). Some teenage girls with T1D develop eating disorders and skip insulin as a way of avoiding weight gain (Daneman et al., 2002). Substance use in parents or adolescents can create upset and inattention to self-care. Changing Jim's diabetes treatment without involving him and his mother with a mental health professional is unlikely to be effective if they have mental health needs that are unaddressed.

What about Autonomy?

Autonomy, the freedom to make one's own choices, is a sensitive issue with adolescents. One of life's tasks during adolescence is to "individuate," to develop an individual identity apart from one's family and peers. Yet, minors also live in relationship with parents or caregivers who are legally responsible for their actions, health, and well-being. Good parenting during adolescence is about gradually allowing greater autonomy and emerging freedom of choice while maintaining both appropriate limits and a strong loving relationship.

When treating adolescents who have diabetes, you are managing at least two interrelated care relationships, one with the adolescent and the other with the parent(s). Fortunately, MI can be useful in dealing with both relationships. First, older adolescents respond well to MI themselves (Naar-King & Suarez, 2011). Second, MI is valuable in encouraging parents to be actively engaged with diabetes care and do whatever is necessary to promote their teenager's

> When treating adolescents who have diabetes, you are managing at least two interrelated care relationships, one with the adolescent and the other with the parent(s).

health and safety. An authoritative parenting role walks the delicate line between being either overcontrolling or underengaged. A parent who takes a heavy-handed approach in forcing diabetes care or does too much for the teen both invites pushback and undermines the teen's learning the self-management skills that are needed in adulthood. On the other hand, poor self-care of diabetes is a nearly inevitable result if parents are disengaged from ensuring that the adolescent does what is so important for his or her current and future health. In essence, the authoritative middle road parallels the very same guiding style of MI.

In areas unrelated to diabetes, parents can usually communicate clearly with their teenagers about their expectations for certain behaviors. If a behavioral expectation is not met, a reasonable consequence ensues—for example, the loss of driving privileges for a reasonable interval of time if seat belts are not used. These expectations are common in areas like school attendance, driving, substance use, and dating. However, parents often hesitate or do not even think of combining behavioral expectations and brief periods of losing privileges when their teenagers repeatedly ignore essential aspects of diabetes self-care.

In the following interview MI is combined with a behavioral management approach to help adolescents and their families improve glycemic control. Keep in mind that in most of pediatric health care the patient is not just the adolescent. Both the parents and the teenager are the patient. MI is used to discuss and present the behavioral management, an approach that combines both positive incentives for improving diabetes self-care or the loss of a privilege for 3 or 4 days when diabetes self-care is neglected. The treatment provides an incremental approach for achieving improvements in self-care.

This is the first visit for 16-year-old Julia and her parents with a nurse who is also a diabetes educator. Julia has had T1D for most of her life—since she was 7 years old. The diabetes educator has skills in MI. She works exclusively with families, especially those who have adolescents and/or children with diabetes. The family was referred to her by Julia's pediatric endocrinologist. For several years Julia's A1c level has been on the rise, her most recent reading being 11.5%. Julia makes good grades in school, is on the basketball team, and is well liked by her teachers and her many friends.

NURSE EDUCATOR: Hello, Julia. Your doctor sent referral information to me but I'd like to know your reason for coming here today. (Open question)

JULIA: My A1c is 11.5%, and my parents and doctor wanted me to talk to you.

NURSE EDUCATOR: Your A1c is high and your family and doctor are concerned about it. (Simple reflection)

JULIA: There's been a lot going on about this.

NURSE EDUCATOR: You've gotten a lot of attention from others, and you're feeling pressure about it. (Complex reflection that ends with a guess)

JULIA: Yeah.

NURSE EDUCATOR: The information your doctor sent says you have a lot of friends and are active at school. You get good grades and are good at basketball. (Affirmations)

JULIA: Yeah.

MOTHER: This problem has been going on over a long time. When we go to the doctor's office, we find out she checks her blood glucose less than 2 or 3 times a day. When the doctor looked at the report from her pump this time, she had skipped insulin at lunchtime almost all of the time.

NURSE EDUCATOR: It sounds like Julia likes school and does well in it, yet the care for diabetes seems to be on a vacation. (Reflection)

FATHER: That's the truth. For the past 5 years we've been struggling with her to get diabetes care going. She's seen diabetes educators, who have pretty much given up on her. One of them regularly texted her for weeks to remind her about checking her blood glucose and giving insulin before she eats. When she asked about whether Julia had given insulin for a recent meal, there was usually no response at all from Julia.

JULIA: My parents have no idea of what it's like to have diabetes.

MOTHER: That's not true. You and I worked together so well when you were younger. You should know by now that we are really concerned about you—not just about your diabetes, either. We had good relationships until you became a teenager.

NURSE EDUCATOR: (looking at Julia) Julia, you think your parents don't understand your diabetes. (looking at the parents) Both of you think Julia can do better with her diabetes; that's something you want to see. Each of you is having a difficult time because Julia doesn't want to take care of her diabetes.

JULIA: Right. My parents nag me all of the time about diabetes. We argue about it a lot. I hate all that stuff!

FATHER: We have to keep after you to get anything to happen with your diabetes. You know how to take care of yourself. We wouldn't need to be talking to you about diabetes all the time if you took care of it. She refuses to listen to us about her diabetes.

MOTHER: She knows that we want her to check her blood glucose levels before meals and snacks and give herself a dose of insulin for food and for her blood glucose if it's too high. We taught her how to do this stuff years ago.

NURSE EDUCATOR: Your mother and father are really frustrated by the way you care for your diabetes. You'd like your parents to stop nagging you. (Simple reflection) What do you think all this fuss is about, Julia? (Evoking)

JULIA: It bothers them that I'm forgetting stuff about my diabetes.

NURSE EDUCATOR: What do you think about that situation? (Evoking)

JULIA: I don't know . . . I'm pretty forgetful about it. They don't like my A1c being so high.

NURSE EDUCATOR: What do you think about your A1c? (Evoking)

JULIA: I'd like it to be better. (Change talk—desire) Anybody would want that.

NURSE EDUCATOR: You're right about elevated A1c levels being a problem. (Affirmation) You have some concerns about it too. (A reflection that makes a guess)

JULIA: Yeah, I would like it to be lower.

NURSE EDUCATOR: How would you go about doing that? (Evoking)

JULIA: I don't know . . . I just don't remember my diabetes at school or when I'm having a good time with friends.

MOTHER: It's not just forgetting . . . I have to stand in front of you or you won't do a blood glucose before supper.

NURSE EDUCATOR: Julia, can you think of any benefits you would have if you decided to take care of your diabetes? (Evoking)

JULIA: My parents would be happier with me. They'd also stop giving me a hard time about it. The doctor is always trying to scare me with those bad things that could happen. He'd be happier too.

NURSE EDUCATOR: You want a lower A1c and you have other good reasons for doing something about your diabetes. Would it be OK with each of you if we talked about other areas of your life, Julia? (Asking permission to expand focusing)

[The parents agree.]

NURSE EDUCATOR: How about you, Julia? Is it OK with you?

JULIA: OK.

NURSE EDUCATOR: I want to understand how your parents establish what's expected of you, Julia. This may sound like a silly example, but it helps me understand how you communicate with one another. Julia, what would happen if you told your parents that you, your boyfriend, and a couple of other friends have been skipping school for the past three school days and you're hanging out at a friend's house whose parents aren't home because you like being there more than being at school? (Evoking with an open question)

JULIA: (*with a large, amused smile*) That's wild. They'd explode if I told them I did that.

NURSE EDUCATOR: It's something you couldn't get away with. Your parents have rules about that kind of behavior. (Simple reflection)

JULIA: They sure do.

NURSE EDUCATOR: (*looking at the parents*) I'm assuming you're thinking Julia wouldn't do what I just suggested. But let's say—just for the fun it—what would happen if she did? (Open question)

JULIA: I'll tell you . . . I'd be in a lot of trouble.

FATHER: That's fair to say.

NURSE EDUCATOR: (*looking at the parents*) Julia knows well that there are rules and consequences for important behaviors in her life. What are your rules about diabetes self-care?

FATHER: I think I know where you're going with this. We've told you what we expect in her care for diabetes.

NURSE EDUCATOR: Good, you've been thinking about the expectations you have about Julia's diabetes. And you do have reasonable expectations, checking blood glucose levels before meals and snacks, the use of insulin for meals and snacks, and corrections of high blood glucose levels when she does her testing. (Affirmation of the father's implied insight) What will it be like for Julia if she continues to ignore her diabetes? (Evoking with an open question)

FATHER: We're all aware of that, including Julia. She'd develop complications from her diabetes.

NURSE EDUCATOR: And you want your daughter to be healthy, and she told me she does too. That's really an important goal for each person in your family. (Complex reflections)

MOTHER: It means a lot to each of us. That's why we're working so hard on this. It's the main reason why we came to see you today.

NURSE EDUCATOR: (*looking at all three people*) Would it be OK if I asked a difficult question about something you may not have considered?

FATHER: Sure.

NURSE EDUCATOR: What about you, Julia.

JULIA: Yeah.

NURSE EDUCATOR: As parents can you think of any way to make the complications of unattended diabetes less severe? (Evoking with an open question)

FATHER: What do you mean? We can't control her diabetes . . . she has to do that.

NURSE EDUCATOR: You're right about that. It is Julia's job to take care of her diabetes, and I believe she could do a good job of it too. (Affirmation) You not only have expectations about school, you also have consequences for not following the rules. You're both reasonable parents too. If she skipped school with her friends, it would likely be a temporary loss of privileges.

FATHER: Going out with her boyfriend wouldn't happen for a while in the example you just described. . . . But how could something like that be done with her diabetes? It's bad enough to have it. She doesn't need to lose privileges because of it.

NURSE EDUCATOR: You have reasonable concerns. And I want to assure you that what you do about this issue with diabetes will be determined by what the three of you decide to do, not by me. (Respecting the patient's autonomy) I can offer each of you some ideas if it would be helpful.

FATHER: I want to hear what you have to say.

MOTHER: I do too.

NURSE EDUCATOR: Julia, what about you?

JULIA: I'm not sure what you're going to say, but go ahead.

NURSE EDUCATOR: All of you are concerned about this issue. (Complex reflection) This is one way, Julia, that you could get rid of all the nagging. What do you think about that?

JULIA: That sounds great to me.

NURSE EDUCATOR: To accomplish that, Julia, you could perhaps make a deal with your parents to review your diabetes for just 10 or 15 minutes twice a week. What do you think about that?

JULIA: I don't know what it would involve.

FATHER: I'm not sure either. What does it involve?

MOTHER: I'm not sure I can stop talking about her diabetes with her when she's at home. If it weren't for me, she would hardly ever check her blood glucose levels.

NURSE EDUCATOR: (*looking at the father*) You asked what this involves; it's pretty simple. The three of you would review Julia's diabetes together twice a week for 10 to 15 minutes to see if the basic diabetes care has been done—checking blood glucose levels at least 4 times a day, before each meal and at bedtime, and administering insulin for each meal or snack. (*looking at Julia*) If you did this review, Julia, I suspect your parents would agree not to nag you any more about it. You are an accomplished person, Julia, you have a history of doing things well. (Affirmation) What do each of you think about this? (Evoking)

FATHER: How could we tell those things are being done?

NURSE EDUCATOR: By downloading her insulin pump and meter onto your computer, you can all review the results.

FATHER: That's right! I've never thought about that.

MOTHER: Neither had I.

NURSE EDUCATOR: If Julia meets the minimum expectations of four blood glucose tests and provides insulin for meals and snacks she could receive a reward. If she doesn't there will be a 3- or 4-day loss of a privilege.

JULIA: I feel like all of this is my business, not theirs.

NURSE EDUCATOR: You're concerned about reviewing your self-care for diabetes. That's understandable. However, all three of you already know what's going on.

JULIA: I guess so.

MOTHER: We'd be able to see what's going on before the doctor does. (Preparatory change talk—reasons) And we could talk together with Julia. (Preparatory change talk—desire)

FATHER: Knowing what's going on would help us understand the situation better. (Preparatory change talk, reasons)

JULIA: I'd love it if I wasn't being nagged all the time. (Preparatory change talk, desire) What about the rewards?

FATHER: If she didn't take care of her diabetes what would we do?

NURSE EDUCATOR: That's up to you. You've done a good job helping Julia with school and social behaviors. (*looking at the parents*) All three of you indicated an interest in avoiding complications. You as parents (*looking at them*) could offer a reasonable reward and if Julia didn't test and use insulin she would lose a privilege until the next review in 3 or 4 days. However, she would have her privileges intact in addition to a reward if she met the expectations. It's similar to what you do now in other areas. What do each of you think?

MOTHER: We need to do something! (Different preparatory change talk—need) What we're doing now isn't working. (Preparatory change talk—reason)

FATHER: That's true. It might help all of us. (Preparatory change talk—reason)

JULIA: I don't know. I'm not interested in losing privileges. I'd like to think I could avoid that by doing all this stuff (Preparatory change talk—ability) but I might not be able to. (Ambivalence) What would the reward be?

NURSE EDUCATOR: The reward is up to your parents and you. I hear some interest in this from each of you. What are your thoughts about trying this? (Reflection followed by open question addressing commitment)

FATHER: It's worth a try as it is. All three of us will discuss it. Julia is the most important person in this. I think she will work with us and, we can work with her. This idea could help us. Nothing else we've tried has worked so far.

MOTHER: It's going to be hard for me not to talk with her about these things during the week.

JULIA: Mom, give me a break! I've had diabetes for 9 years. I know how to do this stuff!

MOTHER: You don't want me to help you refill your pump with insulin and help you remember when to change your infusion site?

JULIA: Let me do it!

NURSE EDUCATOR: You've worked out a plan. Would it be helpful to demonstrate how to download the pump and the meter? (Asking permission to provide information)

FATHER: We can manage that.

NURSE EDUCATOR: When would you like to follow up?

MOTHER: Sooner rather than later.

NURSE EDUCATOR: Most families who are just starting this come back in two weeks.

MOTHER: We'll make an appointment before we leave.

It is often more difficult to work with parents in this area than it is to work with their teenager. Understandably, it is difficult for them. They may feel sorry or responsible for their child's diabetes and cannot smoothly transition age-appropriate diabetes self-care responsibilities to their developing son or daughter. Also, diabetes can be quite stressful for parents: they know all about diabetic complications and feel helpless if they cannot easily influence the way their teenager is taking care of his or her diabetes. The enormous commitment of time and energy to help children and adolescents achieve better outcomes can also exert a negative influence on the parents' quality of life (Whittemore et al., 2012).

Unfortunately, history has shown us that debilitating diabetic complications are just as great a risk, if not greater, to the health and well-being of adolescents as are other risky areas previously mentioned. The nurse educator engaged with the family by using reflections, open questions, and affirmations in her discussion with them. She also did not push a solution on to them. In the latter half of the interview, she emphasized respect for the autonomy of all three of them. The nurse educator used the heartset of MI well. She took time to develop a partnership with Julia and her parents. Her acceptance of them was evidenced by her attitude and affirmations. She evoked their experiences and was compassionately focused on their current and future welfare.

Most parents have expectations as their children become adolescents that age-appropriate diabetes self-care will be maintained by them. Our lives in childhood and adulthood are in part defined by what we expect of ourselves and also what others expect of us. However, in the struggles of adolescence to achieve independence, the motivation of teenagers with T1D often wanes, and the difficult work leading to better diabetes outcomes falls away. It is appropriate for anyone with diabetes to dislike having it. It is also appropriate for parents to help their teenagers learn that there is a huge benefit provided by taking good care of it. This approach includes small, desirable rewards for achievements in self-care, things like a music download or a small financial incentive. The immediate consequence of briefly losing a privilege can be lamentable for teenagers; however, it pales significantly in comparison to the benefit of better health and diabetes outcomes in adulthood.

Key Points

- Parents of adolescents play key roles in facilitating diabetes self-care activities by clearly creating realistic expectations and reviewing progress on a weekly/regular basis. Ideally, self-care activities in adolescence are part of a process moving forward from the age of diagnosis and into adolescence.

- In working with adolescents, "the patient" is the family. Having parents and adolescents at appointments creates a diabetes counseling opportunity involving each individual.

- MI skills—focusing, evoking, and reflective listening—fit well into diabetes care with families and adolescents with T1D.

- Respect for autonomy provides an opportunity for people to think and then make decisions about what they want. It avoids discord and creates a person- or family-centered experience.

CHAPTER 16

Managing Diabetes-Related Complications

Diabetes-related complications are dreaded, and unfortunately they occur all too frequently. For people with diabetes, their families, and their health care clinicians, complications are challenging to care for. Most of them are caused by the long-term metabolic disruptions that diabetes creates. The complications occur in two areas of the body's arterial circulation, in small arteries (microvascular circulation) and large ones (macrovascular circulation).

Microvascular complications are related to both the magnitude and duration of hyperglycemia and the presence of hypertension. Microvascular injury from proliferative or nonproliferative retinopathy is the most common microvascular complication. Proliferative retinopathy occurs when small new arteries appear in the retina in response to decreased retinal oxygen levels. The new arteries grow into the posterior chamber of the eye that is filled with vitreous humor, a gel-like material. The presence of new vessels and the bleeding they cause lead to approximately 10,000 new cases of blindness annually in the United States (Fong, Aiello, Ferris, & Klein, 2004). Nonproliferative retinopathy, also known as background diabetic retinopathy, is more indolent and treatable. It is caused by microaneurysms in the small retinal arteries behind and on the surface of the retina. This disorder responds to laser treatment when microaneurysms break and leak blood into the retina. However, sometimes it becomes unresponsive to treatment and can then progress to proliferative retinopathy.

An important study provided good news about eye complications. In T1D, improved glycemic control in combination with ophthalmologic treatment can improve outcomes in the early stages of nonproliferative retinopathy (Diabetes Control and Complications Trial Research Group, 1993). It took 2 years of improved glycemic control to create an impact on outcomes. To emphasize the value of ophthalmologic screening and glycemic control, eye physicians report their findings to the patient's physician, nurse practitioner, or physician assistant when they perform annually recommended eye exams for people with diabetes.

Hypertension and hyperglycemia damage small arteries in the kidney, another site of microvascular complications. This leads to the loss of protein in urine (proteinuria) and marks the early stage of diabetic nephropathy. It can progress to end-stage renal disease, necessitating dialysis and/or a kidney transplant. Forty percent of people with T1D and T2D have diabetic nephropathy, the urinary loss of over 0.5 grams of protein daily (Gross et al., 2005).

Damage to peripheral nerves (those outside of the brain and spinal cord) is another microvascular complication. It can affect sensory (most commonly), motor, and/or autonomic nerves. This is also a common diabetic complication, occurring in about 50% of all people with diabetes (Tesfaye et al., 2010). In the feet, sensory neuropathy can result in the loss of protective sensation, creating the risk that minor foot injuries go unnoticed. These foot injuries often become infected ulcers that may lead to lower limb amputations.

Atherosclerosis is the main cause of macrovascular complications, myocardial infarctions, strokes, and peripheral arterial disease, primarily presenting as decreased circulation in the lower extremities. Heart disease (primarily myocardial infarction), the leading cause for death among people with diabetes, was mentioned on 68% of the death certificates for people with diabetes in 2004 (Centers for Disease Control and Prevention, 2011a, p. 8).

One group of complications occurs acutely, hyperglycemic crises—of which there are two types, diabetic ketoacidosis (DKA) and hyperosmolar hyperglycemic state (HHS). DKA occurs after deprivation of insulin and is usually present when T1D is diagnosed. Although some cases of DKA occur in people with T2D, DKA is much more frequently encountered in people with T1D. HHS is predominantly a disorder of T2D that occurs in the context of major stressors like infection, strokes, and myocardial infarctions. These hyperglycemic crises are emergencies that cause death if left untreated.

There is good news about the U.S. incidence rates for diabetic complications. In the 20-year period from 1990 to 2010, percentage declines in incidence rates were sizable—67.8% for myocardial infarction, 52.7% for stroke, 51.4% for amputation, 28.3% for end-stage renal disease, and 64.4% for death from hyperglycemic crisis (Gregg et al., 2014).

The percentage of people between 1997 and 2011 with visual impairment not correctable with glasses or contact lenses (who are likely to have diabetic retinopathy) also decreased by 27% (Centers for Disease Control and Prevention, 2012a). Some people without vision impairment have diabetic retinopathy that has not progressed to the point of impaired vision. The number of people with diabetes who had visual impairment in 2011 was 4.0 million (Centers for Disease Control and Prevention, 2012b).

The upbeat news of declines in the percentage of people with diabetic complications is significant. The news reflects valuable improvements in diabetes care and outcomes, nonetheless the number of people actually suffering from at least one of the conditions has dramatically increased. However, during the 20-year span that incidence rates dropped, the total burden of people with diabetes rose significantly from 6.5 million in 1990 to 20.7 million in 2010 (Gregg et al., 2014). During that period of time, many effective new drugs were introduced. Additionally, technologies used mostly in T1D—insulin pumps, continuous glucose monitoring, and the increased use of self-managed blood glucose testing—have facilitated improved diabetes self-care.

> *During the 20-year span that incidence rates dropped, the total burden of people with diabetes rose significantly from 6.5 million in 1990 to 20.7 million in 2010.*

Despite the improved options for diabetes treatment and the declining rates of complications, the total number of adults with diabetes in the United States experiencing acute myocardial infarction, stroke, amputation, end-stage renal disease, or death by hyperglycemic crises increased substantially, from 338,155 in 1990 to 448,087 in 2010 (Gregg et al., 2014).

Life with Complications

The longer one has diabetes, the greater the likelihood of complications. Of the 25.8 million people in the United States with diabetes, an estimated 7 million remain undiagnosed (Centers for Disease Control and Prevention, 2011a, p. 1). Unfortunately, some of the people who are undiagnosed do not find out they have diabetes until a diabetes-related complication is discovered. For example, diabetes is unexpectedly found when people present with myocardial infarctions or strokes, or at eye exams, or in laboratory tests when retinopathy or kidney disease is discovered.

Adding to the challenges of life with complications is the fact that a single complication places people at higher risk for other complications. Microvascular complications increase the risks of myocardial infarctions and strokes. Macrovascular complications are risk factors for diabetic retinopathy and nephropathy.

For people with diabetes, the occurrence of complications is viewed by some as a failure of self-management. Many people who have struggled with self-care improvements are aware of the publicity created by studies demonstrating that diabetes complications can be delayed or avoided by a combination of good health care and a personal dedication to self-care (Diabetes Control and Complications Trial Research Group, 1993; UKPDS Study Group, 1998).

Diabetes-related complications are replete with experiences that trigger stress and/or depression (deGroot, Anderson, Freedland, Clouse, & Lustman, 2001), adding significantly to the challenges of diabetes self-care. People with diabetes have more appointments with health care professionals and with those who provide social support and mental health care than people without diabetes. Also a new list of self-care tasks filled with what to do or not to do accompany the condition(s) as soon as the diagnostic evaluation is completed. Fitness for work can be affected. Expenses escalate significantly.

Knowing that depression or stress can become a further complication within these complications, can help you offer better care to your patients. Depression frequently accompanies diabetes complications (Gendelman et al., 2009; Hedayati et al., 2009; Kinder et al., 2006). Bringing it up at each patient visit is appropriate. The PHQ-9 is more than a screening tool for depression. Scores from it can be easily used at subsequent visits to gauge if treatment for depression is adequate or not (see Chapter 13) (Kroenke et al., 2001). The cornerstones of the spirit of MI—partnership, compassion, acceptance, and evocation—are well suited to conversations centered on the difficult decisions and treatments that people with complications endure.

> *The cornerstones of the spirit of MI—partnership, compassion, acceptance, and evocation—are well suited to conversations centered on the difficult decisions and treatments that people with complications endure.*

Ed, the 66-year-old man in the following interview, is at an appointment with his nurse case manager. He had a myocardial infarction 18 months earlier that resulted in chronic congestive heart failure. He is currently able to slowly walk the distance of one city block before stopping to rest. He dresses himself, drives to appointments, and cooks the meals at home for his wife and himself during her workweek. She does all of the shopping. He has had T2D for 19 years. This appointment was occasioned by his third hospitalization in 8 months for congestive heart failure. Myocardial infarctions resulting in heart failure significantly increase the risk of death for people with diabetes (Domanski et al., 2003). Ed's history of recurrent hospitalizations is concerning.

The following interview begins after the case manager and Ed have reviewed his long list of medications and records of his daily weights, used to determine the daily dosing of his diuretic medication. If his weight gain from fluid retention exceeds 2 pounds daily, he takes an additional dose of the diuretic. The case manager has just asked Ed about other daily activities.

ED: I walk about a block and then back again on the sidewalk in front of my house three or four times a day. And a friend or two comes by about once a month. If it weren't for my dog, I'd be real lonely during the week when my wife's at work.

CASE MANAGER: It's good that you're walking several times a day. (Affirmation) During the week you'd like to spend more time with people. (Simple reflection)

ED: The people I worked with was the reason I enjoyed my work so much. We became friends outside of work. I still really like them. Before my heart attack, every weekend I spent time with my friends. And I'd often go out with my wife on Friday night. I feel like a loner now. Life wasn't like this before the heart attack.

CASE MANAGER: Being with friends makes your life more enjoyable. You feel down without them. (Empathy and complex reflections)

ED: I feel down because I can't do a lot of things I used to be able to do. And I miss my friends. The medicine for depression doesn't talk or play cards with me. It helped when I started it a couple of years ago, but not so much recently. That's why Dr. Smith put me on that new one.

CASE MANAGER: You know that taking the new medicine is something valuable for your depression. (Affirmation) What would you have to do to get more time with your friends? (Open question—evoking his ideas)

ED: I don't know. Nowadays it's hard for me to get things going. It's not like it was before all this happened.

CASE MANAGER: A few months ago you were seeing your friends more frequently. But before this hospitalization something happened, and you stopped seeing them.

ED: I was driving to their houses occasionally, and sometimes one of them would pick me up and we'd play bridge or watch a game on TV. But I felt bad when I was alone. And then I slowed down with some of my pills. First, the medicine for depression. I didn't stop it completely, but I took it less. I also stopped some of my heart medicines before I was hospitalized. I felt like all I was doing was taking pills.

CASE MANAGER: Your doctor told you it was important to take the medications. (Intended as a reflection, but Ed responds forcefully as if it were a confrontation)

ED: I get it! You'll spend the rest of the time I'm here lecturing me about the pills so I don't end up back in the hospital.

CASE MANAGER: I'm sorry . . . I wasn't trying to gang up on you with your doctor. (Avoiding discord with an apology followed by an empathic statement) I didn't say that well. I was just wondering if your depression caused most of what's going on now, stopping the medicines and the visits with friends and then your hospitalization. I was hoping that depression was a topic of discussion during the hospitalization. (A reflection that guesses)

ED: In the hospital they just wanted to get me out quickly. Everybody's so busy. The hospital doctor gave me a tough time about not taking my medicines. When I saw Dr. Smith last week, he wanted to talk about that too. (Frustration) The nurses were lots nicer, even though they were real busy too. One of them asked me about depression. It got me thinking about how I was feeling before I got admitted . . . not too good.

CASE MANAGER: The nurse understood you. And that helped you think about how your depression was influencing you. (Both reflections involve guesses)

ED: Yeah . . . but it's not something I feel good about. It's no fun being in the hospital. (Change talk)

CASE MANAGER: What would help you stay out of the hospital in the future?

ED: The pills were a big part of all of this.

CASE MANAGER: That makes sense. Your depression got worse and that might have been part of what led to your being hospitalized, which is something you don't like. (Complex reflection)

ED: Maybe so.

CASE MANAGER: I'm glad you're trying a new medication, and I have another idea that I can offer if that's OK with you.

ED: Sure.

CASE MANAGER: You used to drive yourself to your friends' houses to play cards in the evenings just a few months ago, and you miss that. Being isolated can make depression worse, and I wonder how you might get back into going to see your friends. (Evoking)

ED: Once you quit doing something, it's not easy to start it up again. (Sustain talk) I don't know what my friends would think about me.

Maybe I could talk with the psychologist again. (Change talk—"able") She understood the whole picture . . . how all of this has been for me. It did help me to see her. (Change talk—"reasons")

CASE MANAGER: That sounds like a good idea. (Affirmation of the change talk) How would you go about doing that? (Evoking)

ED: I have the phone number for her office. I'll call her. (Mobilizing change talk)

CASE MANAGER: When do you think you could do that? (Open question)

ED: I need to get out of the house. She helped me before. I'll do it this week. (Need and reasons . . . with more mobilizing change talk)

CASE MANAGER: That's a good idea. And you're trying the new medication for depression as well.

ED: Look, I'm already taking nine medicines a day, some of them a couple of times a day. It's not something I enjoy. When the doctor suggested a different antidepressant last week, I told him I would try it. It hasn't bothered me so far.

CASE MANAGER: Good, you've taken a big step toward improving your depression. (Affirmation) Can you think of anything else that you could do to ease your depression? (Evoking)

ED: I'd like to see my friends. You caught me when you said I could get back into visiting my friends, but I don't know if I can do it. (Ambivalence)

CASE MANAGER: You really enjoy being with your friends. Their companionship is important to you.

ED: Right. I can talk with Mary about that when I see her. (Change talk—ability) It's often hard for me to get going. (Sustain talk)

CASE MANAGER: I'd like to summarize what we've talked about. You want to get back together with your friends in the evening. And you made a plan for working with Mary, your psychologist, to help you with this and the depression. You are going to call her for an appointment. When you saw Dr. Smith, you decided to start a new antidepressant and are taking it daily. Even though you don't enjoy taking medications, you know they help you, especially the ones for heart failure. (Reflective summary)

ED: I'm also seeing Dr. Smith for my diabetes and the medical stuff next week.

CASE MANAGER: I know it takes a lot to take care of yourself—all these medications and appointments—and I'm glad you're being so persistent! (Affirmation) If it's all right with you, I will call you weekly, and you can call me too if something comes up. Does that sound all right? (Seeking permission for phone follow-up)

ED: Sure.

MI in Difficult Settings

People who use MI in their practices often report that it makes their work easier and more enjoyable. Having skills to work with more complex patients is valuable to many clinicians. Rather than being faced by needs to be persuasive or insistent, practitioners using MI have conversations that help people by evoking their ideas and plans. It is a sharp contrast to the righting reflex, the burdensome experience of trying to "make" people change when they are overwhelmed and struggling. That situation is frequently seen in diabetes-related complications.

Rather than being a technique, MI is more a style for having conversations that combine evidence-based counseling skills with a specific "mind and heart," the spirit of MI. In the preceding interview, the case manager relied heavily on evocation, eliciting Ed's own feelings and ideas with reflective listening and open questions. Empathy was present in many of her complex reflections.

When Ed took offense at her comment about medications, she responded with an apology and empathy to reengage. Rather than taking an expert stance, she "wondered" about depression contributing to his difficulties. The conversation that began with empathy, partnership, acceptance, and evocation continued. Ed offered preparatory and mobilizing change talk as they discussed a plan. Ambivalence was still present. He complained a few times about how difficult it was to do things, a conspicuous feature of depression. Instead of focusing on the ambivalence, the case manager expressed what Ed wanted in her complex reflections, "You enjoy being with your friends. Their companionship is important to you." He did not resolve his ambivalence but instead made a helpful decision to discuss it with the psychologist.

Key Points

- The cornerstones of the spirit of MI—partnership, compassion, acceptance, and evocation—fit well in conversations centered on the difficult decisions and treatments that people with complications face.

- MI skills help practitioners work with people in medically complex situations. Evoking people's ideas about various treatment options helps them to build plans, through the complexities, toward what they want to do.

- Offering an apology when patients are offended by what was said avoids discord and facilitates further discussion.

- People with diabetic complications have higher rates of depression and stress. It is appropriate to discuss this topic during each visit.

PART III

LEARNING AND APPLYING MOTIVATIONAL INTERVIEWING

CHAPTER 17

Learning Motivational Interviewing

There is good news about the process of learning MI. First, it is learnable! Studies of MI training show substantial strengthening of practitioners' skills over time. The ability to learn MI seems unrelated to the number of years of graduate education or to one's advanced degrees (Miller et al., 2004). Even early in implementing MI, practitioners often report noticeable differences in their patients' responses. And, as described in Part I, once you know what to listen for, your patients become your teachers. When you offer a complex reflection making a guess about what someone means, you get immediate feedback that over time helps you to make more accurate guesses and reflections in the future. When practicing MI, hearing change talk represents immediate feedback that you're doing something right. When you hear defensiveness or a lot of sustain talk, that's your patient telling you to try something different. Such immediate feedback allows you to learn, just as it does in the practice of surgery: surgeons who have performed a procedure a thousand times are simply better at it than they were in their first operation.

What this means, of course, is that it takes some time to become skillful in MI. Be patient with yourself; it's like learning any other complex skill. Sometimes clinicians come to our workshops expecting to learn MI in an afternoon, as if it were a simple trick or technique. Unfortunately it's not as simple as "see one, do one, teach one." MI is more like a practice style—not particular words so much as a way of conversing with patients about change. As a musician develops a distinctive personal sound, clinicians find the MI style that works best for them. There is no one right way of doing MI, and, as in health care more generally, it is your patients' responses that tell you when you're on the right track.

How to Get Started

Reading about MI can help you understand what it involves, and there are plenty of written materials available as well as video resources available from a wide variety of practitioners demonstrating MI (at *www.motivationalinterviewing.org*). We've done our best to provide in this book a concise overview and practical examples for those who work in diabetes care. As with many medical procedures, reading and watching is only a beginning and is unlikely in itself to yield proficiency.

Training workshops are available at various skill levels in most of the United States and in at least 30 other countries (see *www.motivationalinterviewing.org/motivational-interviewing-training*). Such workshops should include ample opportunities to practice component skills, ideally with some feedback from a skilled MI practitioner. Participants in such workshops on average show a significant, albeit modest increase in practice skills (Madson, Loignon, & Lane, 2009). A prodigious minority do demonstrate reasonable competence in MI after a workshop, but for most clinicians additional learning opportunities are needed to develop enough skillfulness to make a difference for their patients (e.g., Miller et al., 2004).

Continuing to Learn

There are at least two additional aids in learning any complex skill: feedback and coaching. First, you need reliable information about how you're doing. One could take online knowledge tests for years, but very little learning will occur unless there is feedback about correct and incorrect responses. You won't improve your golf or tennis swing much if it is pitch black and you can't see where the ball goes, and it's hard to become proficient in playing an electronic keyboard with the power switch turned off.

Feedback requires listening to practice. One doesn't hire a piano teacher and say, "But don't listen to me—I'd be too embarrassed," or a golf coach and say, "But don't watch me." We learned long ago that, when students come out of a consultation and tell us what happened, it's often what they *didn't* see and hear that is important.

Even listening to your own practice can be instructive. You can hear things that you were too busy to notice during the consultation. Obviously, this requires some recording of practice so that you (or a coach) can review it later. The idea of having one's practice recorded and reviewed can be surprisingly intimidating, even though observed practice is how health care professionals normally learn their craft during training. Just give it a try. Most clinicians focus on their patients and quickly forget that they are being recorded. We find that an audio recording is usually sufficient and tends to be less daunting than video, for patient and practitioner alike.

(Recording requires your patients' formal, written permission, of course, with a clear explanation of how the recording will be used and protected and when it will be destroyed.)

The value of reviewing recorded practice with patients is that it can help you learn and improve your skills. In listening to your own practice you can, for example, count reflections and questions. We recommend in MI practice that reflections should at least outnumber questions. Were your questions open-ended or closed, and how did the patient respond to each? What change talk did you hear, and what did you do just before it that may have prompted the change talk? If the patient began backing away from change with sustain talk or defensiveness, what preceded that?

It can also be useful to get feedback from a knowledgeable coach who listens to your practice. This can be done as you talk to a "standardized patient," an actor simulating a clinical encounter with you, but we find that such actors seldom respond the same way real patients do. Actual patients, for example, tend to offer more change talk in response to MI-consistent practice, whereas actors are more likely to stick to a developed role and are not as responsive to different clinician styles. So, a coach can be most helpful to you by listening to samples of your normal clinical practice of MI.

Developing proficiency in MI involves learning and integrating a set of component skills (Miller & Moyers, 2006). A good coach will not list 14 things to do differently next time, but he or she will comment on what you are already doing well and then suggest one or two practical changes to try. Skillful coaching involves understanding where the person is in skill development at present and knowing what would be a useful next step.

A Sequence of Skills

MI does involve learning and integrating several complex skills. While there is no fixed order in which to develop practice proficiency, in this section we revisit some of the component skills.

The Spirit of MI

As discussed in Chapter 2, the practice of MI is facilitated by a particular mindset—thinking of patients as capable partners and collaborators in change. In a way, MI is a negotiation process, moving toward a plan for change that is acceptable and feasible. MI starts by accepting rather than judging, and it proceeds by evoking rather than providing solutions. This "spirit" is not a prerequisite for the

> *MI starts by accepting rather than judging, and it proceeds by evoking rather than providing solutions.*

practice of MI, but it does serve as a framework for understanding what you are doing and why.

Reflective Listening

Reflective listening (described in Chapter 4) is a foundational skill for practicing MI, and thus it is one to hone early. At first, the forming of reflections can feel awkward. It seems much easier just to ask questions. Yet, it is nearly impossible to practice MI without good reflective listening. Intentional practice of reflection represents a good investment of your time, and because you receive immediate feedback each time you reflect, your skill and comfort level grow over time.

Focusing

Having a clear change focus (discussed in Chapter 3) is another helpful discipline. Consultation conversations can easily get off track, and with limited time it is important to keep in mind where you intend to go. As the Cheshire cat observed in *Alice in Wonderland*, if you don't know where you're going, any road will take you there. Develop a clear change goal. What is the next healthy change step for this patient? Remember that focusing is a process of negotiation, not prescription.

Exchanging Information

The collaborative elicit–provide–elicit (E-P-E) way of exchanging information is a skill that can be practiced within minutes (as described in Chapter 6). Instead of simply dumping information on your patients, start by *asking*. Ask for permission. Ask what the patient already knows. Ask what the patient would like to know. Then provide a manageable chunk of information or advice, and again ask for the patient's response to what you have said, following with reflection.

Change Talk

It is a skill just to know change talk when you hear it. So often change talk flows by in a consultation without the practitioner recognizing or responding to it! Know that change talk is of particular importance when what you are striving for is behavior change on the part of your patient.

Once you can recognize change talk, the next step is to try to evoke it (see Chapter 5). What open question could you ask that might elicit change talk? As with reflections, you get immediate feedback every time you try this.

A third skill here is how to respond to change talk. When you hear change talk, don't just sit there. What should you say next to invite more change? The OARS acronym—open questions, affirming, reflecting, summarizing—prompts appropriate responses. Responding to change talk is a component skill that can be practiced any time you hear change talk, and once again you receive immediate feedback: Did your response elicit more change talk?

Responding to Sustain Talk and Discord

When you encounter what feels like resistance, how do you respond? Chapter 5 offers a few suggestions to try so that you don't increase sustain talk and discord. Once more, feedback is immediate. If your righting reflex gets tweaked and you fall into making the arguments for change, the patient is likely to give you more sustain talk.

Planning

Another component skill is negotiating a change plan that the patient is willing to implement. What you hope to hear is a next-step implementation intention, a specific plan to which the patient says "Yes," expressing the intention to carry it out. You get feedback during the consultation from the patient's mobilizing change talk, and then in the next visit you ask whether the patient implemented the plan and how it is going. Although most health care visits are relatively brief, it is an advantage if you see patients periodically over time and can renew your use of MI to promote their self-care.

Learning Communities

One way to develop skills is to work with a group of colleagues interested in improving proficiency in MI. In such a group there is often no "MI expert," and instead the task is learning together. This approach might include discussing readings or clinical experiences, watching training videotapes, or taking turns with a "journal club" that presents research articles on MI in health care fields. A variety of structured learning exercises can be used (Rosengren, 2009). A vital component, however, is *observed practice*, which usually means listening to audio recordings of each other's patient consultations. It is important that the atmosphere not be critical (catching what someone did wrong), evaluative, or competitive ("Who's the best?"). Rather, the process is one of puzzling together, sharing ideas, and trying out possibilities: "In this particular patient situation, how might we respond in an MI-consistent way?" We recommend always listening for particularly *good* examples of MI practice and commenting on those.

Members of the group can also use a structured tool in listening to practice samples (Madson & Campbell, 2006). A simple one is to count occurrences and record good examples of each. Each member might listen for a different aspect of practice, such as:

- components of MI spirit (Chapter 2)
- presence of each of the four MI processes (Chapter 3)
- OARS (Chapter 4)
- patient change talk (Chapter 5)

There are also well-developed instruments for rating MI practice quality that can provide reliable measures along with published comparative data (e.g., Hendrickson et al., 2004; Lane et al., 2005; Moyers, Martin, Catley, Harris, & Ahluwalia, 2003).

A key requirement in learning MI is to approach practice (and patients) with an open "beginner's" mind. MI is not about being clever, coming up with the perfect question or reflection. It is about being fully present in the moment, curious to learn about your patient's own wisdom and ideas. It is not just dispensing knowledge and advice but, rather, calling forth that which is already there. Approach your own learning with that same beginner's mind, open to the new experience that each patient brings. MI is a skill set that you can continue to develop throughout your career, and the real beneficiaries will be your patients.

> *MI is about being fully present in the moment, curious to learn about your patient's own wisdom and ideas.*

Key Points

- Developing proficiency in MI involves learning and integrating a set of component skills.

- Reflective listening is a necessary foundational skill in learning and practicing MI.

- Recognizing, evoking, and responding to change talk are also key skills.

- As with any complex skill, individual feedback and coaching based on observed practice can be helpful in learning MI.

- A learning community is a group of colleagues working together to improve their skill.

CHAPTER 18

Motivational Interviewing in Groups

If your practice sometimes includes meeting with patients in groups, this chapter addresses how you can use MI in such consultations. Medication education is typically delivered in groups using a structured curriculum, and group formats can also be effective in diabetes self-care education (Beverly et al., 2013). Some practices offer group medical visits. Seeing patients together for diabetes education or consultation may reduce per-patient cost, and it also offers patients potential motivational benefits through their interactions with you and with each other.

Though MI was originally developed for one-to-one consultations, the same style can be used with groups to strengthen patient motivation for and commitment to change (Wagner & Ingersoll, 2013). Using MI in groups is somewhat more complex, however, because you must attend to the motivational dynamics described in previous chapters while also managing group processes to stay on task. We recommend honing your MI skills first in one-to-one consultations, if possible.

Engaging

As with individual consultations, task number 1 with a group is to engage every participant—to establish an atmosphere of collaboration, empathy, and trust. Even (perhaps especially) if you have a lot of material to cover, spending some initial time in engaging is a good investment. The process can be as simple as asking a few open questions and responding with reflective listening. Because the focus

> *As with individual consultations, task number 1 with a group is to engage every participant.*

205

of the group will often be predetermined (i.e., some aspect of diabetes self-management), the engaging questions that you choose to ask can also be designed from the outset to begin evoking change talk. Here are a few examples:

> "What would you most like to know about diabetes?"
> "Tell me about what steps you are already taking to manage your diabetes."
> "What do you already know about how to stay healthy when you have diabetes?"
> "What are some good reasons to keep your glucose levels well controlled?"

Using questions like these as "ice breakers" can get the discussion moving in a positive direction from the beginning, and are more likely to be helpful and engaging than the usual introductions (name, occupation, and how long you've had diabetes).

The fact that you respond with empathic listening is also important at the outset. It signals that you are interested in your patients' own perspectives and do not respond judgmentally. It encourages patients to be active participants rather than passive recipients—an important difference within an MI perspective.

Giving Information

Diabetes education can be very information heavy. To be sure, there is much to learn, particularly for recently diagnosed patients. The temptation is to download everything that you think people need to know. The pressure to do this is even greater when time is short and you have a required curriculum to cover. It is the group equivalent of the expert-model righting reflex, that is, these people lack knowledge, and I have to install it.

Even if time is short and fact lists loom, keep the elicit–provide–elicit (E-P-E) approach in mind. How possible is it for the session to be more like a conversation than a data dump? Again, it doesn't have to be complicated.

Elicit

Here are three examples of "Elicit" questions to start the E-P-E process.

"What do you already know about _____?"

We find that often patients already have quite a bit of information about diabetes, even if some of it is misinformation. They browse the Internet, talk to friends with diabetes, and pick up reading materials in the doctor's office or pharmacy. There are at least three good reasons to start a topic by asking what patients already know about it.

1. It's boring if not disrespectful to tell people what they already know.
2. Hearing the patients' own words gives you information about how they understand the facts and also where there may be some misunderstanding that you might have missed if you were just lecturing.
3. There is value in having patients themselves give voice to the facts, since people tend to be more persuaded by what they themselves say.

When you ask an open question like "What do you already know?" to a group, there are several important aspects of how you respond. First of all, *listen* to make sure you understand what the person is saying. Respond to him or her positively and respectfully, encouraging others to take part as well. Highlight in your own words whatever correct information is presented. Find at least part of what the person has said that is correct, and add additional information as needed.

LEADER: So, tell me what you already know about checking your sugar level.

PARTICIPANT 1: It hurts! (*laughter*)

LEADER: Yes it does, a bit! Who knows what you can do to minimize any discomfort?

PARTICIPANT 2: I change the lancet pretty often. When it's new you hardly feel it.

LEADER: Good! Do you all know what she's talking about? (*a few head nods*)

PARTICIPANT 2: And you can also change how deep it goes.

LEADER: Right. You already have a lot of experience with testing. (Affirmation)

PARTICIPANT 3: I push the button and then right away focus on getting a drop of blood out and onto the test strip. It takes my mind on to the next thing.

LEADER: I see! Instead of just focusing on the momentary pinprick. Good idea.

The skill is to keep the conversation moving and lively, eliciting the facts that you want to convey from the participants as much as possible.

"What would you most like to know?"

Another opening "elicit" question is to ask what the participants would most like to know. Again respond in a way that encourages people to keep participating actively.

> LEADER: There is a lot we could discuss about changing how you eat, and I'm sure you know some of this already. I don't want to be telling you what you already know. So, tell me this: What would you most like to know about food and diabetes? What would be most helpful for me to talk about?
>
> PARTICIPANT 1: The food labels are confusing. Tell us what we should pay attention to.
>
> LEADER: Good! I'll do that, and also ask some of you what you pay attention to on labels. What else?
>
> PARTICIPANT 2: Can I ever eat fast food?
>
> LEADER: Good question. In this country we eat a lot of meals out. Of course, you *can* do whatever you want, but we could discuss how to eat healthfully in less healthy places.
>
> PARTICIPANT 3: I've heard that carbohydrates are really bad for you when you have diabetes.
>
> LEADER: A really important topic! It's not quite that simple, but we will definitely be talking about carbs.

Asking Motivational Questions

The same MI principle can apply in groups as in individual consultations: Ask open-ended questions the answer to which is change talk. Most likely, the people in your group were not forced to come. They might have reservations, but part of them also wants to be healthy. Early in a session you can ask an open question to evoke change talk about the topic(s) at hand.

> LEADER: Today we're going to talk about physical activity. Some of you already know a lot about this, and I'm sure there are lots of different kinds of activity represented in the room here. So, let's start there. Tell me a little about what kind of physical activity you already enjoy or have enjoyed in the past.
>
> PARTICIPANT 1: I used to really enjoy cross-country skiing in the winter, but with the weight I've gained, that's pretty hard now.
>
> LEADER: I enjoy it, too! It can be such a pleasure to just clip on the skis and head off through the woods—really peaceful.

PARTICIPANT 1: But at least I walk now, and when it's really cold I go to the shopping center before it gets crowded.

LEADER: Good! So, there's one simple kind of activity that really makes a difference. What do you enjoy about it?

PARTICIPANT 1: I like watching the people and seeing what's in the store windows. I take along my music, too.

LEADER: Great! What do others of you do to be active?

PARTICIPANT 2: I go to the gym and use the equipment. Not one of those show-off gyms; it's a "Silver Sneakers" place for seniors where they're really helpful.

LEADER: They show you how to use the equipment safely. (Reflection)

PARTICIPANT 2: And they know my name when I come in.

LEADER: That's a good feeling. What other kinds of activity have you fit into your daily life?

PARTICIPANT 3: I hate going to gyms, but I've got an incline trainer at home, and I listen to music while I exercise.

LEADER: That works! What kind of music do you enjoy?

A lot is happening here. Members of the group are suggesting different kinds of physical activity (much better than your listing them) and are modeling for each other how to fit in physical activity. The leader is encouraging each new idea, expressing interest and curiosity. Some "buddy" relationships may emerge if participants find common interests. Importantly, people are expressing change talk about what they *can* do (ability) and *enjoy* doing or want to do (desire).

All of these are examples of asking before telling (elicit–provide) and of a more Socratic style for eliciting the information that you hope to convey. It doesn't have to take a long time, but resist the thought of getting the questions out of the way so that you can do the really important thing, lecturing!

Provide

The more information exchange that can happen in this conversational manner, the better. Sometimes, though, there is a certain amount of standard information to be covered, and not all of it can be elicited from participants. There may be rubber food to show, test kits to demonstrate, and brochures to distribute. Fair enough.

As described in Chapter 6, a good tip is to present information in small digestible chunks (provide) and then ask for responses (elicit). Rather than didactic lecturing (provide–provide–provide–provide), presenting small amounts of information and then asking for responses retains the interactive E-P-E style that engages people in their own learning. There are many possible elicit questions you can ask after providing a chunk of information:

"What more can I tell you about this that would be helpful?"
"How might you fit this into your daily routine?"
"Give me some examples of how you have done this."
"Does that make sense to you?" (A closed question, but nevertheless useful)
"What do you think about that?"
"Given what you know about yourself, how might you use this idea?"
"Now, you suggest another idea."
"What surprises or concerns were there for you in what I've been saying?"

Evoking

The preceding sections have touched on giving information and engaging as fundamental processes in working with a group. The focus in diabetes groups, we assume, will generally be on behavior and lifestyle changes to promote health and manage glucose levels. But, how does evoking occur in groups? Each participant has limited air time, and if an important motivational task is to evoke change talk, how can that be accomplished in a group?

Round-Robin

One approach is to ask an open question to evoke change talk (as illustrated above) and have participants take turns offering their own responses. In a smaller group this can be done by going around and asking for each person's response. It's good to give participants a "pass" option if they choose not to respond, but most will have something to say. Listen, in particular, for change talk, and reflect it. Keep the discussion moving, and if responses drift away from the topic, focus back on the initial question, such as:

"What works best for you in remembering to take your medications?"
"What for you is the most important reason to exercise?"
"What is one healthy change that you think would be possible for you to make in your daily eating habits?"

In a larger group there is not time to elicit a response from every participant. Invite responses and reply to each in a way that encourages others to speak (e.g., affirm, reflect). Keep the process moving by asking "What else?" Invite a response from individuals who have not been speaking.

Individual Thinking Time

Another way to engage each member of a group is to give all participants a minute or two to think about and write down their own responses to a specific question, such as:

> "What specific changes do you think you could make to manage your diabetes?"
> "Write down three good reasons for you to stay physically active."
> "Which potential complications of diabetes concern you the most?"

Doing this engages each and every group member actively in responding to a topic. It counteracts the temptation to disengage and let others talk. Research on brainstorming also shows that you will get many more ideas from a group if you do this first: have each person list their own ideas before anyone speaks.

Beyond taking group time for individual reflection, it is also possible to give writing assignments to be completed between sessions. If you do this, be sure to take time early in the next session to review what participants have written. Never give an assignment and then ignore it.

Dyads and Triads

With larger groups, another way to encourage active engagement and increase talk time is to have participants break into groups of two or three to discuss a specific topic. It's good to provide a clear structure and a specific time limit to help people keep on task. One option is a sentence completion task:

> "The most important reasons for me to keep my diabetes under control are _____."
> "I want to stay healthy so that in the years ahead I can _____."
> "Three good changes that I could make in my everyday life are _____."
> "What I would most like to have some ideas about is _____."

Planning

The strengthening of motivation is of limited use if it is not channeled into action. Whereas the evoking process focuses on whether and why to change, planning focuses more on how and when. Health behavior change is promoted by a combination of perceived importance and confidence that

_____

The strengthening of motivation is of limited use if it is not channeled into action.

_____

the change is both *needed* and *possible*. Sometimes people with diabetes clearly see the importance of change (e.g., for future health, survival, and quality of life) but lack confidence that they can do it. In fact, people are understandably reluctant to admit that change is important if they believe it is not possible for them. Within any group you may have some people for whom the primary obstacle to change is importance (and for whom the evoking process is needed) and others whose primary challenge is confidence (for whom the planning process is more helpful).

The righting reflex often rears its head when it comes time for planning. After all, you have professional expertise about how to manage diabetes, and it is tempting to just start dispensing knowledge and advice once patients seem motivated enough for change. Much of diabetes education assumes a planning focus ("Here's how to _____."), too often skipping over the prerequisite processes of engaging, focusing, and evoking. Within MI there is a place for offering information and advice, and it is also important (and possible) to maintain an empathic and evoking E-P-E style even during the planning process. Working with groups can make it easier to maintain this balance precisely because there is so much expertise among the patients in the room.

Consider two contrasting educational styles. One is represented by the Latin verb *docere*, an expert-focused insertion model of education. The expert has the knowledge, and he or she needs to install it. In a group format, this takes the form of a lecture to a relatively passive audience. *Docere* is the etymologic root of words like docent, doctrine, indoctrinate, and doctor. A contrasting Latin verb is *educare*—to draw out, as in drawing water from a well. This is a more Socratic, give-and-take, E-P-E style of teaching. Education is not about shoving knowledge in, but together drawing it out.

In essence, we are recommending the same collaborative style when working with a group in the planning process. You have how-to knowledge to share. Patients also bring vital knowledge about themselves and often substantial information (as well as some misinformation) about diabetes. Together you can do the problem solving of how to make the changes that will promote long-term health.

Working from a Menu of Options

One approach with a group is to describe a variety of changes that people with diabetes can make to maintain good health. The descriptions can be brief, like the names of items on a menu. In fact, you could use the group itself to brainstorm such possible changes, perhaps first using the "individual thinking time" approach described above. Think of yourself as the knowledgeable server at a restaurant. People will have questions that you can answer about various items on the menu, and ultimately they are the ones who choose.

With such a list of health behavior options presented (perhaps on a flip chart, board, or slide), you can ask the group what questions they have about the menu, or what each member might "order"—what change(s) would seem most important and possible to implement, given what they know about their lives?

Engaged Planning

In a smaller group you can use an E-P-E style to involve patients in planning how to implement their own health behavior changes. In a round-robin format, people can volunteer what changes seem most possible and practical as next steps in their diabetes self-management, and how they might make those changes, given what they know about themselves. In any sized group, patients can work together in dyads or triads to develop a plan for implementing specific healthy changes.

Implementation Intentions

People are more likely to implement a change if they express to someone else a specific plan for doing so (when, where, how, etc.) and the intention to do it. In a smaller group that meets over time, each participant may voice to the group their specific implementation intention, for example: "This week I am going to [specific action]," with details of when and how. In a larger group, this can be done in dyads or triads.

The most fun I ever had as a diabetes patient was in a group gathered to learn about how to cook for people with diabetes. It was an affordable class offered by a county extension office, and there were about 20 of us, including some spouses who did the cooking at home. We received a lot of useful information in digestible chunks, with plenty of time for discussions and questions. The leaders also welcomed ideas from the group about what we had already learned and tried, what changes had been working for us. Then we broke up into groups to prepare a diabetes-friendly and delicious meal, trying out different foods at each session. We learned not only from the facilitators but from each other, swapping recipes, favorite brands, websites, and practical ideas. We were definitely engaged in the learning process!

—WRM

In the mid-1990s, a diabetes educator working in our office reminded me of a health and wellness week sponsored by the local hospital. She asked if I had any ideas. I was busy and responded without thinking, "Why don't we invite people with diabetes to meet with us at noon on one of the days? We will ask them for topics, and each of us will wing it from there." At the conclusion, it was obvious people had enjoyed themselves. They asked to repeat this format monthly, and both of us agreed, asking them in advance what they would like to hear about. More people attended the second meeting. It went well. When the meeting began, the group wanted to organize themselves. They formed a phone tree to reach one another easily and elected a leader. Over the next 9 years, they became constant positive voices for diabetes in the community. Three or four of them on insulin offered to work with peers starting insulin. They organized an annual lunch meeting as well and named the group "the Diabetes Support Group." All of the leadership came from group members. Our practice grew, and we added a diabetes educator. The three of us were awed by the work of this group. It taught me that a group of people with diabetes on their own can become a strong, vocal community presence.

—MPS

Being Creative with Groups

Though patient groups are common in medication education, we believe that there are many more creative ways in which groups could be used in diabetes care. One possibility is to offer a regular open drop-in discussion time for people with diabetes, perhaps a brown-bag lunch meeting. Such a group may cycle through a set of topics or just have an open discussion format. Patients often appreciate the ability to meet and talk with other people living with diabetes, the flexibility of a drop-in structure, and the ability to ask questions of a knowledgeable professional. Flexible groups of this kind may not generate billable hours but can be offered as a pro bono community service and may help with practice building. Such groups may also be staffed by volunteers with successful experience in diabetes self-management.

Group Medical Visits

Diabetes care delivered in a group medical visit is a wonderful opportunity for using MI. The group context facilitates a variation in guiding. This method for delivering care, of course, involves planning. The group visit can be designed to combine heterogeneous people—some of whom are on target and others who are not—in selected areas of diabetes self-care. Topics for group discussion at the visit focus on the area(s) of heterogeneity within the group. A skillful moderator—a physician, physician assistant, nurse practitioner, or diabetes educator—can evoke comments from different members of the group.

Lively discussions usually take place, with people sharing their approaches to dealing with challenging areas of self-care and others listening quietly on the sideline. Interestingly, group visits occasionally lead to individual visits by patients who realize at the group visit they need to do something different with their diabetes care and would like a private session to discuss it in more detail. The group setting offers peer input and the opportunity for patients to socialize during the appointment.

Group medical visits are billable if they meet the guidelines for medical decision making. This involves determining the medical complexity of the visit based on the number of diagnoses and management options, the amount and complexity of data that were reviewed, and the risk of complications. Additionally, the visits need to include at least two of three elements of an individual appointment: history, physical exam, and/or review of systems. Group visits have been shown to have positive effects on diabetes care, with lower A1c levels (Riley, 2013) and increases in weekly exercise time (Dickman, Pintz, Gold, & Kivlahan, 2012).

Key Points

- MI can be useful when working with groups as well as individuals.
- Task number 1 with any group is to engage every participant.
- Instead of lecturing, use engaging and evoking strategies to encourage active participation of group members.
- Information can be provided in an elicit–provide–elicit style.
- A creative challenge is how to evoke as much change talk as possible from each group member.

CHAPTER 19

Motivational Interviewing, Diabetes Prevention, and the Global Epidemic of Diabetes

A robust epidemic of diabetes is not a future possibility; it is here now. The continually increasing number of people across the globe with prediabetes and T2D is shocking. From a public health perspective, no epidemic can be addressed by treatment alone. A comprehensive approach must also include prevention. Prevention and treatment are complementary endeavors that lie along a single continuum. This chapter focuses on how MI may be useful in such prevention efforts.

> *Prevention and treatment are complementary endeavors that lie along a single continuum.*

Three Levels of Prevention

Three overlapping levels of prevention are recognized in the field of public health. *Primary* or *universal prevention* efforts are typically delivered to whole populations (whether it be a city, school, or workplace) with the intention of reducing the incidence of new cases of a disease. *Secondary* or *selective prevention* targets one or more subgroups of a population known to be at increased risk of developing a disease in the future, though they do not currently meet diagnostic criteria. Finally, *tertiary* or *indicated prevention* focuses on people who already have at least an early form of the disease, with the goal of reducing future severity, complications, and disability. Though conceptually useful, these types of prevention do indeed overlap. If a prevention program targets an entire population known to be at increased risk, it spans the universal and selective domains of prevention. If a program is designed for people with prediabetes, does it represent selective or indicated intervention? The point is that interventions can be designed all along a continuum from the general population to those already diagnosed with a disease, at which point prevention becomes continuous with treatment.

MI was originally developed in the domain of treatment and indicated prevention to reduce the future severity and consequences of a condition like alcohol use disorders (Miller, 1983; Miller, Forcehimes, & Zweben, 2011) where behavior change is key and motivation for change is often a significant clinical issue.

Diabetes Prevention

The increasing number of people at risk for developing diabetes reinforces the argument for developing reliable approaches to reach that goal. Diabetes exacts huge tolls from people who have it. Additionally, from a public health perspective, it imposes enormous expenses on governments and other organizations that pay for its care. For example, in the United States more than one dollar of every five dollars spent on health care pays for the direct and indirect costs of diabetes. The direct costs are the expenses paid to individuals and organizations providing health care for diabetes and its complications. The indirect costs of diabetes include absenteeism and decreased productivity at work, reduced productivity from those not in the workforce, lost productive capacity at work from disabilities due to diabetes complications, and lost productive capacity from the premature mortality of people with diabetes (American Diabetes Association, 2013). Both diabetes prevention programs and improvements in the care for T2D can improve the health of many people.

Lifestyle modifications are the foundation of diabetes prevention programs. MI has been widely used in helping people change challenging areas of their life in the treatment of obesity (Armstrong et al., 2011; Williams, Hollis, Collins, & Morgan, 2014), diabetes prevention (Penn et al., 2009), high-risk adolescent behaviors and substance use disorders (Cleary, Hunt, Matheson, & Walter, 2009; Cushing, Jensen, Miller, & Leffingwell, 2014), and adult substance use disorders (Lundahl & Burke, 2009).

People with prediabetes and/or metabolic syndrome are candidates for targeted prevention. The former group has impaired fasting glucose levels ranging from 101 to 124 mg/dl (5.4 to 7.0 mmol/liter) or A1c levels between 5.7% and 6.4%. These levels are above the normal ranges for blood glucose and A1c, but they are not as high as the diagnostic criteria for diabetes (Centers for Disease Control and Prevention, 2014). Both groups of candidates must also be overweight (BMI > 25 to < 30 kg/m^2) or obese (BMI ≥ 30).

Metabolic syndrome is a group of co-occurring conditions—hypertension, obesity with abdominal adiposity, specific serum lipid abnormalities, and high levels of serum triglycerides and low levels of high-density lipoprotein (HDL) cholesterol (National Institutes of Health, 2011). Prediabetes and metabolic syndrome place people at risk for myocardial infarctions and diabetes that are twofold and fivefold greater, respectively, than for people without those two conditions (Mottillo et al., 2010). There are also many adolescents and children with metabolic syndrome.

Like diabetes, prediabetes has also become an epidemic. A stunning percentage of the world's adult population is at increased risk for T2D, with metabolic syndrome occurring in 25% of the global population (International Diabetes Federation, 2014).

Although there is no known prevention for T1D, three of the first controlled clinical trials in diabetes prevention showed that combinations of lifestyle modifications—weight loss, physical activity, and/or healthy diets—could prevent T2D alone or in concert with metformin, the most common drug used to treat T2D (Diabetes Prevention Program Research Group, 2002; Pan et al., 1997; Tuomilehto et al., 2001).

China, with one of the highest incidences of T2D in the world (Xu, Wang, He, & et al., 2013), was the site for one of the earliest diabetes prevention programs in 1986. Investigators sought to prevent non-insulin-dependent diabetes mellitus, a former term for T2D. The study included 577 people with impaired glucose tolerance, (IGT), known in recent years as prediabetes. Study participants were randomly assigned to a control group or one of three treatment arms—diet alone, exercise alone, or diet plus exercise. The control group received information about diabetes and IGT. The treatment groups received regular counseling and information about the lifestyle modification(s) being used in their group. After 6 years of study, 67.7% of the control group had developed diabetes. The incidence of diabetes in the treatment groups was 43.8% for the diet only group, 41.1% for the exercise only group, and 46% in the diet plus exercise group. The differences between the control group and all of the intervention groups were significant at $p < .05$ (Pan et al., 1997).

The Finnish Diabetes Prevention Study (DPS) also confirmed the viability of T2D prevention (Tuomilehto et al., 2001). The study included men and women with obesity (average BMI of 31) and IGT. The people in the experimental group received personalized counseling focusing on lifestyle modifications. The goals of counseling included weight loss, physical activity, and dietary changes. Specific individualized information was not provided to the control group. Instead, they received generalized information that was written and provided in groups about diet and the appropriate sizing of portions of food. They also had yearly follow-up and completed a 3-day food diary at each of their annual visits. The groups were followed for an average of 3.2 years. At the end of the study, lifestyle modifications for the intervention group resulted in a 58% reduction in the risks of developing T2D. The mean change in weight was significant: a 4.5-kg loss $\pm$ 5.1 kg (mean $\pm$ SD) in the intervention group, compared to 0.8 kg $\pm$ 3.7 in the control group ($p < .001$). In the intervention group, there were significant changes in triglyceride levels, waist circumference, fasting blood glucose levels, and postmeal insulin levels, all at the probability level of $p < .001$. Systolic and diastolic blood pressures also changed in a positive direction, $p < .007$ and $p < .02$, respectively (Tuomilehto et al., 2001).

The first U.S. clinical trial to prevent diabetes published its results a year later. The Diabetes Prevention Program (DPP) involved 3,234 participants and was the largest of the three prevention trials. People were randomly assigned to the intervention group and agreed to engage in physical activity for at least 150 minutes weekly. Second, they agreed to participate in an intensive lifestyle modification program that included recommendations for healthy eating and dietary changes to facilitate weight loss of at least 7%. There were also two other groups of participants. The second group of people consented to take metformin at a dosage similar to that used in the care of T2D, 850 mg twice daily. In the control group participants received a placebo instead of metformin. Over 25 medical centers across the United States followed participants for an average of 2.8 years. The results confirmed once again that T2D could be prevented or delayed. The incidence of T2D (per 100 person-years) in the placebo group was 11.0%, in the metformin group 7.8%, and in the physical activity/lifestyle modification group 4.8%. The average number of people that needed to be treated in order to prevent one case of diabetes was just 6.9 people in the lifestyle prevention group and 13.9 in the metformin group (Diabetes Prevention Program Research Group, 2002).

There are controversies about diabetes prevention. Although prevention or delayed onset of diabetes has been demonstrated in landmark clinical studies, in some less-resourced community-based sites the results have not been as promising (Kahn & Davidson, 2014). However, encouraging results have been obtained in one low-population state that sponsored successful community-based programs in eight locations (Vanderwood et al., 2010).

Understandably, one of the most difficult areas in health care is the challenge of maintaining weight loss. A study that analyzed the DPP reported weight loss had a potent impact on diabetes prevention. Each kilogram of weight loss reduces diabetes risk by 16%. Yet, beginning in the second year, people began to regain weight (Hamman et al., 2006). Nonetheless, in the 10-year follow-up report on the original DPP participants there were favorable outcomes among all three groups. When the study was unmasked, participants in the metformin placebo group could start metformin, and all three groups had the opportunity to attend group education sessions. After 5–7 years of access to that protocol, all three treatment groups had similar incidences of diabetes, 4.9–5.9 per 100 person-years. It is estimated that original and later metformin groups delayed the onset of diabetes by 4 and

2 years, respectively (Knowler et al., 2009). In the 5-year follow-up report, there were no differences in the incidences of cardiovascular complications among the groups. It was suggested, then, that the 3-year time interval is probably too short (Ratner et al., 2005). So, follow-up will continue into the future to determine whether other valuable goals are achieved, especially delays in the onset of macrovascular and microvascular diabetic complications in the people who develop diabetes (see Chapter 16).

The ponderous questions about facilitating continued weight loss and continual participation in prevention programs warrant more study. The prevention program studies enrolled only people who professed that they were ready, willing, and able to participate in the programs. All people in health care know, the avoidable outcomes of obesity, prediabetes, and T2D occur far more frequently in the people who are not ready, willing, or able to participate in the way program participants did at the outset of most of the prevention studies. These people may have unresolved ambivalence about diabetes self-care or other conditions that create obstacles not only to self-care but to other critical areas of their life. This is the subpopulation of people with diabetes who struggle with poverty, mental illness, or other pernicious problems. One group in the United Kingdom and Europe, used MI as the way of working with participants in their study (Penn et al., 2009).

Diabetes prevention is a ripe area for comparing MI to the current approaches for facilitating change. This sort of research can suggest new ways to operate diabetes prevention programs. More importantly, it may be useful precisely for those people who are less initially motivated to make health behavior changes.

The Big Epidemic

The increase in people with diabetes in record numbers is occurring in all countries across the planet. This disorder of insulin resistance, T2D, is related to many factors, but a single outstanding factor and the most common example of malnourishment, obesity, is propelling this number forward each year. The epidemic is occurring in developing and developed nations alike. The vast majority of the increase is in new cases of T2D, but T1D is also increasing at a lower rate. In 2013, the International Diabetes Federation reported that there were 382 million people with diabetes worldwide. In China and India alone, there are 163.5 million people with diabetes. The federation also projected that by 2035 the global tally of people with diabetes would be 592 million (International Diabetes Federation, 2013, pp. 11–13).

The demanding work involved in caring for the large number of people diagnosed with diabetes could overwhelm both resourced and under-resourced locations. The demands continue to grow not only because the number of people with T2D is growing. There are also large numbers of people with undiagnosed T2D, 176 million people (International Diabetes Federation, 2013, p. 11), who are all at an increased risk of developing serious disabilities from a disorder they do not even know they have. When they present at underresourced sites with diabetic complications, the number of premature but avoidable disabilities and deaths will also grow. It is difficult to imagine so many patients struggling with undiagnosed diabetic symptoms, let alone those who are diagnosed and also struggling with the necessary skills to care for their diabetes.

Diabetes practitioners who can competently work with patients to help them develop effective self-care plans need help from others to address the growing demands for diabetes care. Fortunately, work has been done already to prepare the way for paraprofessionals who can use MI. Social support from peers to facilitate insulin use in T2D has been shown to significantly lower A1c levels. The lowering of A1c was related to an increased frequency of insulin use. This was greater in people who engaged in more telephone conversations with peer support (Piette, Resnicow, Choi, & Heisler, 2013).

> *Fortunately, work has been done already to prepare the way for paraprofessionals who can use MI.*

Body and Soul was a collaborative effort to improve fruit and vegetable intake by African Americans. It used volunteer community workers and a health-related volunteer agency to provide research-based interventions to facilitate healthier diets. Significant dietary changes occurred in the treatment group of the study, reflecting a lower intake of fat and an increased intake of fruit and vegetables (Resnicow et al., 2002). A study in India engaged community volunteers in underresourced locations to serve as lay therapists counseling people with alcohol dependency and severe depression. In the preparation for their work, the lay therapists were trained to use MI in their counseling. The study demonstrated the acceptance of the lay therapists. Additionally, assessments of the counseling skills of individual lay therapists by experts and their peers had high levels of agreement (Singla et al., 2014). These studies need to be supported by additional research. They have tentatively concluded paraprofessionals can be used to facilitate behavior change, especially in underresourced settings. This approach could potentially enhance the health care of people with diabetes. Paraprofessionals working with collaborative teams of diabetes practitioners could provide a behavioral skill set to supportively work with people who are facing the burdensome tasks of diabetes self-care or the challenges posed by diabetic complications.

Capable diabetes care involves a host of knowledge and skills. The improvements that have been made in diabetes care in recent years are notable. Effective medications are more widely available, and there is stronger research supporting the numerous options available to enhance the health care of people with diabetes. Just as important, however, are the choices individual health care practitioners make to hone skills for helping people initiate changes to improve their diabetes self-care.

Health care delivery today is gathering momentum in the areas of wellness, prevention, and the care of chronic conditions, especially those disorders like diabetes that are associated with avoidable complications. Because of resource availability, this momentum is found more in developed countries. However, developing countries are well aware of the same need. They are discussing, planning, and identifying resources that could be used in underresourced settings. A skillful capacity to use MI skills is one of these resources. MI provides clinicians with the ability to work with both people interested in wellness and prevention and people struggling with their self-care for a chronic condition.

In the same way health care has been improved over the past 15-plus years by clinical practice guidelines, so can clinicians develop crucial clinical skills to help people change as they work on preventing diabetes and providing good care for it. The use of effective medications, healthy eating habits, and participation in physical activity offers a healthy lifestyle to people with prediabetes and diabetes. Over time, outcomes are influenced by the work diabetes professionals do with their patients. However, people with prediabetes or diabetes hold a stronger hand in determining what happens. The decisions to develop skills for preventing or taking care of diabetes are ultimately a strong force in determining their courses. The skillful behaviors they use are the crucial ingredients for improving outcomes. With your competent care, patients can resolve their ambivalence in the challenging areas and collaboratively develop with you *their own* effective plans for taking care of *their* diabetes or the work they are doing to prevent it.

Key Points

- Diabetes prevention is a ripe area for comparing MI to the current approaches for facilitating change.

- The demanding work involved in caring for the large number of people diagnosed with diabetes could overwhelm both resourced and underresourced locations.

- In the same way that health care has been improved over the past 15-plus years by clinical practice guidelines, so can clinicians develop crucial clinical skills to help people change as they work on preventing diabetes and providing good care for it.

APPENDIX

Systematic and Meta-Analytic Reviews of Motivational Interviewing

Apodaca, T. R., & Longabaugh, R. (2009). Mechanisms of change in motivational interviewing: A review and preliminary evaluation of the evidence. *Addiction, 104,* 705–715.

Armstrong, M. J., Mottershead, R. A., Ronksley, P. E., Sigal, R. J., Campbell, T. S., & Hemmelgarn, B. R. (2011). Motivational interviewing to improve weight loss in overweight and/or obese patients: A systematic review and meta-analysis of randomized clinical trials. *Obesity Reviews, 12*(9), 709–723.

Burke, B. L., Arkowitz, H., & Menchola, M. (2003). The efficacy of motivational interviewing: A meta-analysis of controlled clinical trials. *Journal of Consulting and Clinical Psychology, 71,* 843–861.

Burke, B. L., Dunn, C. W., Atkins, D. C., & Phelps, J. S. (2004). The emerging evidence base for motivational interviewing: A meta-analytic and qualitative inquiry. *Journal of Cognitive Psychotherapy: An International Quarterly, 18*(4), 309–322.

Cushing, C. C., Jensen, C. D., Miller, M. B., & Leffingwell, T. R. (2014). Meta-analysis of motivational interviewing for adolescent health behavior: Efficacy beyond substance use. *Journal of Consulting and Clinical Psychology, 82*(6), 1212–1218.

Daeppen, J. (2008). A meta-analysis of brief alcohol interventions in emergency departments: Few answers, many questions. *Addiction, 103*(3), 377–378.

DiRosa, L. C. (2010). *Motivational interviewing to treat overweight/obesity: A meta-analysis of relevant research.* Unpublished doctoral dissertation, Wilmington University, New Castle, DE.

Dunn, C., Deroo, L., & Rivara, F. P. (2001). The use of brief interventions adapted from motivational interviewing across behavioral domains: A systematic review. *Addiction, 96,* 1725–1742.

Erickson, S. J., Gerstle, M., & Feldstein, S. W. (2005). Brief interventions and motivational interviewing with children, adolescents, and their parents in pediatric health settings: A review. *Archives of Pediatrics and Adolescent Medicine, 159,* 1173–1180.

Heckman, C. J., Egleston, B. L., & Hofmann, M. T. (2010). Efficacy of motivational interviewing for smokng cessation: A systematic review and meta-analysis. *Tobacco Control, 19*(5), 410–416.

Hettema, J. E., & Hendricks, P. S. (2010). Motivational interviewing for smoking cessation: A meta-analytic review. *Journal of Consulting and Clinical Psychology, 78*(6), 868–884.

Hettema, J., Steele, J., & Miller, W. R. (2005). Motivational interviewing. *Annual Review of Clinical Psychology, 1*, 91–111.

Hill, S., & Kavookjian, J. (2012). Motivational interviewing as a behavioral intervention to increase HAART adherence in patients who are HIV-positive: A systematic review of the literature. *AIDS Care: Psychological and Sociomedical Aspects of AIDS/HIV, 24*(5), 583–592.

Ismail, K., Winkley, K., & Rabe-Hesketh, S. (2004). Systematic review and meta-analysis of randomised controlled trials of psychological interventions to improve glycaemic control in patients with type 2 diabetes. *The Lancet, 363*(9421), 1589–1597.

Jensen, C. D., Cushing, C. C., Aylward, B. S., Craig, J. T., Sorell, D. M., & Steele, R. G. (2011). Effectiveness of motivational interviewing interventions for adolescent substance use behavior change: A meta-analytic review. *Journal of Consulting and Clinical Psychology, 79*(4), 433–440.

Knight, K. M., McGowan, L., Dickens, C., & Bundy, C. (2010). A systematic review of motivational interviewing in physical health care settings. *British Journal of Health Psychology, 11*(2), 319–332.

Lai, D. T. C., Cahill, K., Qin, Y., & Tang, J-L. (2010). Motivational interviewing for smoking cessation. *Cochrane Database of Systematic Reviews* (1), CD006936.

Lundahl, B., & Burke, B. L. (2009). The effectiveness and applicability of motivational interviewing: A practice-friendly review of four meta-analyses. *Journal of Clinical Psychology, 65*(11), 1232–1245.

Lundahl, B., Moleni, T., Burke, B. L., Butters, R., Tollefson, D., Butler, C., et al. (2013). Motivational interviewing in medical care settings: A systematic review and meta-analysis of randomized controlled trials. *Patient Education and Counseling, 93*(2), 157–168.

Lundahl, B. W., Kunz, C., Brownell, C., Tollefson, D., & Burke, B. L. (2010). A meta-analysis of motivational interviewing: Twenty-five years of empirical studies. *Research on Social Work Practice, 20*(2), 137–160.

Macdonald, P., Hibbs, R., Corfield, F., & Treasure, J. (2012). The use of motivational interviewing in eating disorders: A systematic review. *Psychiatry Research, 200*(1), 1–11.

Madson, M. B., Loignon, A. C., & Lane, C. (2009). Training in motivational interviewing: A systematic review. *Journal of Substance Abuse Treatment, 36*, 101–109.

Magill, M., Gaume, J., Apodaca, T. R., Walthers, J., Mastroleo, N. R., Borsari, B., et al. (in press). The technical hypothesis of motivational interviewing: A meta-analysis of MI's key causal model. *Journal of Consulting and Clinical Psychology.*

Martins, R. K., & McNeil, D. W. (2009). Review of motivational interviewing in promoting health behaviors. *Clinical Psychology Review, 29*, 283–293.

McGrane, N., Galvin, R., Cusack, T., & Stokes, E. (in press). Addition of motivational interventions to exercise and traditional physical therapy: A review and meta-analysis. *Physiotherapy.*

McMurran, M. (2009). Motivational interviewing with offenders: A systematic review. *Legal and Criminological Psychology, 14,* 83–100.

Miller, W. R., & Wilbourne, P. L. (2002). Mesa Grande: A methodological analysis of clinical trials of treatments for alcohol use disorders. *Addiction, 97,* 265–277.

Miller, W. R., Wilbourne, P. L., & Hettema, J. E. (2003). What works? A summary of alcohol treatment outcome research. In R. K. Hester & W. R. Miller (Eds.), *Handbook of alcoholism treatment approaches: Effective alternatives* (3rd ed., pp. 13–63). Boston: Allyn & Bacon.

Moyer, A., Finney, J. W., Swearingen, C. E., & Vergun, P. (2002). Brief interventions for alcohol problems: A meta-analytic review of controlled investigations in treatment-seeking and non-treatment-seeking populations. *Addiction, 97*(3), 279–292.

O'Halloran, P. D., Blackstock, F., Shields, N., Holland, A., Iles, R., Kingsley, M., et al. (2014). Motivational interviewing to increase physical activity in people with chronic health conditions: A systematic review and meta-analysis. *Clinical Rehabilitation, 28*(2), 1159–1171.

Osborn, L. D. (2007). A meta-analysis of controlled clinical trials of the efficacy of motivational interviewing in a dual-diagnosis population. 67, ProQuest Information & Learning, US. Retrieved from *http://libproxy.unm.edu/login?url=http:// search.ebscohost.com/login.aspx?direct=true&db=psyh&AN=2007-99006- 281&login.asp&site=ehost-live&scope=site.* (Available from EBSCOhost psyh database)

Resnicow, K., Davis, R., & Rollnick, S. (2006). Motivational interviewing for pediatric obesity: Conceptual issues and evidence review. *Journal of the American Dietetic Association, 106*(12), 2024–2033.

Rubak, S., Sandbaek, A., Lauritzen, T., & Christensen, B. (2005). Motivational interviewing: A systematic review and meta-analysis. *British Journal of General Practice, 55,* 305–312.

Schwalbe, C. S., Oh, H. Y., & Zweben, A. (in press). Sustaining motivational interviewing: A meta-analysis of training studies. *Addiction.*

Söderlund, L. L., Madson, M. B., Rubak, S., & Nilsen, P. (2011). A systematic review of motivational interviewing training for general health care practitioners. *Patient Education and Counseling, 84*(1), 16–26.

Thompson, D. R., Chair, S. Y., Chan, S. W., Astin, F., Davison, D. P., & Ski, C. F. (2011). Motivational interviewing: A useful approach to improving cardiovascular health? *Journal of Clinical Nursing, 20*(9–10), 1236–1244.

Vasilaki, E. I., Hosier, S. G., & Cox, W. M. (2006). The efficacy of motivational interviewing as a brief intervention for excessive drinking: A meta-analytic review. *Alcohol and Alcoholism, 41*(3), 328–335.

Wilk, A. I., Jensen, N. W., & Havighurst, T. C. (1997). Meta-analysis of randomized control trials addressing brief interventions in heavy alcohol drinkers. *Journal of General Internal Medicine, 12*(5), 274–283.

References

American Academy of Pediatrics. (2014). Ages and stages: Stages of adolescence. Retrieved from *www.healthychildren.org/English/ages-stages/teen/Pages/Stages-of-Adolescence.aspx.*

American Association of Clinical Endocrinologists. (2013). AACE comprehensive management algorithm 2013. Retrieved from *www.aace.com/files/aace_algorithm.pdf.*

AHA Scientific Statement. (2013). Circulation. Retrieved from *http://circ.ahajournals.org/content/100/10/1134.full.*

American Diabetes Association. (2013). Economic costs of diabetes in the U.S. in 2012. *Diabetes Care, 36*(4), 1033–1046.

American Diabetes Association. (2014). Clinical practice recommendations 2014. *Diabetes Care, 37*(Suppl. 1).

Amrhein, P. C., Miller, W. R., Yahne, C. E., Palmer, M., & Fulcher, L. (2003). Client commitment language during motivational interviewing predicts drug use outcomes. *Journal of Consulting and Clinical Psychology, 71*, 862–878.

Anderson, R. J., Freedland, K. E., Clouse, R. E., & Lustman, P. J. (2001). The prevalence of co-morbid depression in adults with diabetes: A meta-analysis. *Diabetes Care, 24*(6), 1069–1078.

Armstrong, M. J., Mottershead, R. A., Ronksley, P. E., Sigal, R. J., Campbell, T. S., & Hemmelgarn, B. R. (2011). Motivational interviewing to improve weight loss in overweight and/or obese patients: A systematic review and meta-analysis of randomized clinical trials. *Obesity Reviews, 12*(9), 709–723.

Babor, T. F., McRee, B. G., Kassebaum, P. A., Grimaldi, P. L., Ahmed, K., & Bray, J. (2007). Screening, Brief Intervention, and Referral to Treatment (SBIRT): Toward a public health approach to the management of substance abuse. *Substance Abuse, 28*(3), 7–30.

Bao, Y., Duan, N., & Fox, S. A. (2006). Is some provider advice on smoking cessation better than no advice? An instrumental variable analysis of the 2001 National Health Interview Survey. *Health Services Research, 41*(6), 2114–2135.

Barnett, E., Moyers, T. B., Sussman, S., Smith, C., Rohrbach, L. A., Sun, P., et al. (2014). From counselor skill to decreased marijuana use: Does change talk matter? *Journal of Substance Abuse Treatment, 46*(4), 498–505.

Becker, G. (2006). *The first year: Type 2 diabetes: An essential guide for the newly diagnosed* (2nd ed.). Boston: Da Capo Press.

Bernstein, E., Edwards, E., Dorfman, D., Heeren, T., Bliss, C., & Bernstein, J. (2009). Screening and brief intervention to reduce marijuana use among youth and young adults in a pediatric emergency department. *Academic Emergency Medicine, 16*(11), 1174–1185.

Bernstein, J., Bernstein, E., Tassiopoulos, K., Heeren, T., Levenson, S., & Hingson, R. (2005). Brief motivational intervention at a clinic visit reduces cocaine and heroin use. *Drug and Alcohol Dependence, 77*, 497–559.

Bertholet, N., Faouzi, M., Gmel, G., Gaume, J., & Daeppen, J. B. (2010). Change talk sequence during brief motivational intervention, towards or away from drinking. *Addiction, 105*, 2106–2112.

Beverly, E. A., Fitzgerald, S. M., Brooks, K. M., Hultgren, B. A., Ganda, O. P., Munshi, M., et al. (2013). Impact of reinforcement of diabetes self-care on poorly controlled diabetes: A randomized controlled trial. *Diabetes Educator, 39*(4), 504–514.

Brown, M. T., & Bussell, J. K. (2011). Medication adherence: WHO cares? *Mayo Clinic Proceedings, 86*(4), 304–314.

Butwicka, A., Frisen, L., Almqvist, C., Zethelius, B., Lichtenstein, P. (2015). Risks of psychiatric disorders and suicide attempts in children and adolescents with type 1 diabetes: A population-based cohort study. *Diabetes Care, 38*(3), 453–459.

Cameron, F. J., Northam, E. A., Ambler, G. R., & Daneman, D. (2007). Routine psychological screening in youth with type 1 diabetes and their parents: A notion whose time has come? *Diabetes Care, 30*(10), 2716–2724.

Casagrande, S. S., Fradkin, J. E., Saydah, S. H., Rust, K. F., & Cowie, C. C. (2013). The prevalence of meeting A1c, blood pressure, and LDL goals among people with diabetes, 1988–2010. *Diabetes Care, 36*(8), 2272–2279.

Centers for Disease Control and Prevention. (2011a). National Diabetes Fact Sheet, 2011. Retrieved from *www.cdc.gov/diabetes/pubs/pdf/ndfs_2011*.

Centers for Disease Control and Prevention. (2011b). National diabetes statistics 2011. Retrieved from *http://diabetes.niddk.nih.gov/dm/pubs/statistics/#Deaths*.

Centers for Disease Control and Prevention. (2012a). Crude and age-adjusted percentage of adults aged 18 years or older with diagnosed diabetes reporting visual impairment, United States, 1997–2011. Retrieved April 16, 2014, from *www.cdc.gov/diabetes/statistics/visual/fig2.htm*.

Centers for Disease Control and Prevention. (2012b). Number (in millions) of adults aged 18 years or older with diagnosed diabetes reporting visual impairment, United States, 1997–2011. Retrieved April 16, 2014, from *www.cdc.gov/diabetes/statistics/visual/fig1.htm*.

Centers for Disease Control and Prevention. (2012c, November 6). Diabetes data and trends. Retrieved from *www.cdc.gov/diabetes/statistics/complications_national.htm#1*.

Centers for Disease Control and Prevention. (2014). National Diabetes Prevention Program. Retrieved from *www.cdc.gov/diabetes/prevention/factsheet.htm*.

Channon, S. J., Huws-Thomas, M. V., Rollnick, S., Hood, K., Cannings-John, R. L., Rogers, C., et al. (2007). A multicenter randomized controlled trial of motivational interviewing in teenagers with diabetes. *Diabetes Care, 30*(6), 1390–1395.

Chaoyang, L., Ford, E. S., Guixiang, Z., Bakkuz, L. S., & Mokdad, A. H. (2010). Undertreatment of mental health problems in adults diagnosed with diabetes and serious psychological stress: The Behavioral Risk Factor Surveillance System, 2007. *Diabetes Care, 33*, 1061–1064.

Cialdini, R. B. (2007). *Influence: The psychology of persuasion.* New York: Collins Business.

Cleary, M., Hunt, G. E., Matheson, S., & Walter, G. (2009). Psychosocial treatments for people with co-occurring severe mental illness and substance misuse: Systematic review. *Journal of Advanced Nursing, 65*(2), 238–258.

Cramer, J. (2004). A systematic review of adherence with medications for diabetes. *Diabetes Care, 27*(5), 1218–1224.

Cushing, C. C., Jensen, C. D., Miller, M. B., & Leffingwell, T. R. (2014). Meta-analysis of motivational interviewing for adolescent health behavior: Efficacy beyond substance use. *Journal of Consulting and Clinical Psychology, 82*(6), 1212–1218.

D'Amico, E. J., Miles, J., Stern, S. A., & Meredith, L. S. (2008). Brief motivational interviewing for teens at risk of substance use consequences: A randomized pilot study in a primary care clinic. *Journal of Substance Abuse Treatment, 35*(1), 53–61.

Daneman, D., Rodin, G., Jones, J., Colton, P., Rydall, A., Maharaj, S., et al. (2002). Eating disorders in adolescent girls and young adult women with type 1 diabetes. *Diabetes Spectrum, 15*(2), 83–105.

deGroot, M., Anderson, R., Freedland, K. E., Clouse, R. E., & Lustman, P. J. (2001). Association of depression and diabetes complications: A meta-analysis. *Psychosomatic Medicine, 63*, 619–630.

Diabetes Control and Complications Trial Research Group. (1993). The effect of intensive treatment of diabetes on the development and progression of long-term complications in insulin-dependent diabetes mellitus. *New England Journal of Medicine, 329*, 977–986.

Diabetes Prevention Program Research Group. (2002). Reduction in the incidence of type 2 diabetes with lifestyle intervention or metformin. *New England Journal of Medicine, 346*(6), 393–403.

Dickman, K., Pintz, C., Gold, K., & Kivlahan, C. (2012). Behavior changes in patients with diabetes and hypertension after experiencing shared medical appointments. *Journal of the American Academy of Nurse Practitioners, 24*(1), 43–51.

Domanski, M., Krause-Steinrauf, H., Deedwania, P., Follmann, D., Ghali, J. K., Gilbert, E., et al. (2003). The effect of diabetes on outcomes of patients with advanced heart failure in the BEST trial. *Journal of the American College of Cardiology, 42*(5), 914–922.

Dragan, A., & Akhtar-Danesh, N. (2007). Relation between body mass index and depression: A structural equation modeling approach. *BMC Medical Research Methodology, 7*, 17.

Druss, B. G., Rosenheck, R. A., & Sledge, W. H. (2000). Health and disability costs of depressive illness in a major U.S. corporation. *American Journal of*

Psychiatry, 157(8), 1274–1278. Retrieved from *http://journals.psychiatryon-line.org/article.aspx?articleid=174268.*

Egan, G. (2013). *The skilled helper: A problem-management and opportunity-development approach to helping* (10th ed.). Belmont, CA: Brooks/Cole, Cengage Learning.

Fisher, L., Chesla, C. A., Skaff, M. M., Mullan, J. T., & Kanter, R. A. (2002). Depression and anxiety among partners of European-American and Latino patients with type 2 diabetes. *Diabetes Care, 25*(9), 1565–1570.

Fong, D. S., Aiello, L. P., Ferris, F. L., & Klein, R. (2004). Diabetic retinopathy. *Diabetes Care, 27*(10), 2540–2553.

Gakidou, M., Mallinger, L., Abbott-Klafter, J., Guerrero, R., Villalpando, S., Ridaura, R. L., et al. (2011). Management of diabetes and associated cardiovascular risk factors in seven countries: A comparison of data from national health examination surveys. *Bulletin of the World Health Organization, 89*(3), 172–183.

Gendelman, N., Snell-Bergeon, J. K., McFann, K., Kinney, G., Paul Wadja, R., Bishop, F., et al. (2009). Prevalence and correlates of depression in individuals with and without type 1 diabetes. *Diabetes Care, 32*(4), 575–579.

Glynn, L. H., & Moyers, T. B. (2010). Chasing change talk: The clinician's role in evoking client language about change. *Journal of Substance Abuse Treatment, 39*, 65–70.

Golden, S. H., Lazo, M., Carnethon, M., Bertoni, A. G., Schreiner, P. J., Diez Roux, A. V., et al. (2008). Examining a bidirectional association between depressive symptoms and diabetes. *Journal of the American Medical Association, 299*(23), 2751–2759.

Gollwitzer, P. M. (1999). Implementation intentions: Simple effects of simple plans. *American Psychologist, 54*, 493–503.

Gordon, T., & Edwards, W. S. (1997). *Making the patient your partner: Communication skills for doctors and other caregivers.* New York: Auburn House.

Gregg, E. W., Li, Y., Wang, J., Burrows, N. R., Ali, M. K., Rolka, D., et al. (2014). Changes in diabetes-related complications in the United States, 1990–2010. *New England Journal of Medicine, 370*, 1514–1523.

Grimshaw, G., & Stanton, A. (2010). Tobacco cessation interventions for young people. *Cochrane Database of Systematic Reviews, 4*, CD003289.

Gross, J. L., de Azevedo, M. J., Silveiro, S. P., Canani, L. H., Caramori, M. L., & Zelmanovitz, T. (2005). Diabetic nephropathy: Diagnosis, prevention, and treatment. *Diabetes Care, 28*(1), 164–176.

Hamman, R. F., Wing, R. R., Edelstein, S. L., Lachin, J. M., Bray, G. A., Delahanty, L., et al. (2006). Effect of weight loss with lifestyle intervention on risk of diabetes. *Diabetes Care, 29*(9), 2102–2107.

Hamrin, V., & McGuiness, T. M. (2013). Motivational interviewing: A tool for increasing psychotropic medication adherence for youth. *Journal of Psychosocial Nursing and Mental Health Services, 51*(6), 15–18.

Handmaker, N. S., Miller, W. R., & Manicke, M. (1999). Findings of a pilot study of motivational interviewing with pregnant drinkers. *Journal of Studies on Alcohol, 60*, 285–287.

Haugstvedt, A., Wentzel-Larsen, T., Rokne, B., & Graue, M. (2011). Psychosocial family factors and glycemic control among children aged 1–15 years with type 1 diabetes: A population-based survey. *BMC Pediatrics, 11*, 118.

Hedayati, S. S., Minhajuddin, A. T., Toto, R. D., Morris, D. W., & Rush, A. J. (2009). Prevalence of major depressive episode in CKD. *American Journal of Kidney Disease, 54*(3), 424–432.

Hendrickson, S. M. L., Martin, T., Manuel, J. K., Christopher, P. J., Thiedeman, T., & Moyers, T. B. (2004). Assessing reliability of the Motivational Interviewing Treatment Integrity behavioral coding system under limited range. *Alcoholism: Clinical and Experimental Research, 28*(5), 74A.

Hettema, J., Steele, J., & Miller, W. R. (2005). Motivational interviewing. *Annual Review of Clinical Psychology, 1*, 91–111.

Hibbard, J. H., Mahoney, E. R., Stock, R., & Tusler, M. (2007). Do increases in patient activation result in improved self-management behaviors? *Health Services Research, 42*(4), 1443–1463.

Hill, S., & Kavookjian, J. (2012). Motivational interviewing as a behavioral intervention to increase HAART adherence in patients who are HIV-positive: A systematic review of the literature. *AIDS Care, 24*(5), 583–592.

Hoey, H., Aanstoot, H.-J., Chiarelli, F., Daneman, D., Danne, T., Dorchy, H., et al. (2001). Good metabolic control is associated with better quality of life in 2,101 adolescents with type 1 diabetes. *Diabetes Care, 24*(11), 1923–1928.

Holbrook, T. L., Barrett-Connor, E., & Wingard, D. L. (1990). A prospective population-based study of alcohol use and non-insulin-dependent diabetes mellitus. *American Journal of Epidemiology, 132*(5), 902–909.

Howard, A. A., Amsten, J. H., & Gourevitch, M. N. (2004). Effect of alcohol consumption on diabetes mellitus: A systematic review. *Annals of Internal Medicine, 140*, 211–219.

Huang, Y., Wei, X., Wu, T., Chen, R., & Guo, A. (2013). Collaborative care for patients with depression and diabetes mellitus: A systematic review and meta-analysis. *BMC Psychiatry, 13*, 260.

Hudson, D. L., Karter, A. J., Fernandez, A., Parker, M., Adams, A. S., Schillinger, D., et al. (2013). Differences in the clinical recognition of depression in diabetes patients: The Diabetes Study of Northern California (DISTANCE). *American Journal of Managed Care, 19*(5), 344–352.

International Diabetes Federation. (2013). IDF diabetes atlas. Retrieved from *www.idf.org/diabetesatlas*.

International Diabetes Federation. (2014). IDF definition of the metabolic syndrome: Frequently asked questions. Retrieved July 20, 2014, from *www.idf.org/metabolic-syndrome/faqs#three*.

Jensen, C. D., Cushing, C. C., Aylward, B. S., Craig, J. T., Sorell, D. M., & Steele, R. G. (2011). Effectiveness of motivational interviewing interventions for adolescent substance use behavior change: A meta-analytic review. *Journal of Consulting and Clinical Psychology, 79*(4), 433–440.

Kahn, R., & Davidson, M. B. (2014). The reality of type 2 diabetes prevention. *Diabetes Care, 37*(4), 943–949.

Kanny, D., Liu, Y., Brewer, R. D., & Lu, H. (2013). Binge drinking: United States, 2011. *Morbidity and Mortality Weekly Report Supplements, 62*(3), 77–80.

Kaplan, J. E., Keeley, R. D., Engel, M., Emsermann, C., & Brody, D. (2013).

Aspects of patient and clinician language predict adherence to antidepressant medication. *Journal of the American Board of Family Medicine, 26*(4), 409–420.

Karlsen, B., Oftedal, B., & Bru, E. (2012). The relationship between clinical indicators, coping styles, perceived support and diabetes-related distress among adults with type 2 diabetes. *Journal of Advanced Nursing, 68*(2), 391–401.

Katon, W. (2009). The impact of depression on workplace functioning and disability costs. *American Journal of Managed Care, 15*(11, Suppl.), S322–S327.

Kinder, L. S., Katon, W. J., Ludman, E., Russo, J., Simon, G., Lin, E. H., et al. (2006). Improving depression care in patients with diabetes and multiple complications. *Journal of General Internal Medicine, 21*(10), 1036–1041.

King, B. A., Dube, S. R., & Tynan, M. A. (2012). Current tobacco use among adults in the United States: Findings from the National Adult Tobacco Survey. *American Journal of Public Heath, 102*(11), 93–100.

King, P. S., Berg, C. A., Butner, J., Butler, J. M., & Wiebe, D. J. (2014). Longitudinal trajectories of parental involvement in type 1 diabetes and adolescents' adherence. *Health Psychology, 33*(5), 424–432.

Knowler, W. C., Fowler, S. E., Hamman, R. F., Christophi, C. A., Hoffman, H. J., Brenneman, A. T., et al. (2009). 10-year follow-up of diabetes incidence and weight loss in the Diabetes Prevention Program Outcomes Study. *Lancet, 374*(9702), 1677–1686.

Koppes, L. L. J., Dekker, J. M., Hendriks, H. F. J., Bouter, L. M., & Heine, R. J. (2005). Moderate alcohol consumption lowers the risk of type 2 diabetes: A meta-analysis of prospective observational studies. *Diabetes Care, 28*(3), 719–725.

Kroenke, K., Spitzer, R. L., & Williams, J. B. (Producer). (2001, September). The PHQ-9: Validity of a brief depression severity measure. *Journal of General Internal Medicine, 66*(9), 606–613.

Lai, D. T. C., Cahill, K., Qin, Y., & Tang, J.-L. (2010). Motivational interviewing for smoking cessation. *Cochrane Database of Systematic Reviews* (1), CD006936.

Lancaster, T., & Stead, L. F. (2004). Physician advice for smoking cessation. *Cochrane Database of Systematic Reviews* (4), CD000165.

Lane, C., Huws-Thomas, M., Hood, K., Rollnick, S., Edwards, K., & Robling, M. (2005). Measuring adaptations of motivational interviewing: The development and validation of the behavior change counseling index (BECCI). *Patient Education and Counseling, 56*, 166–173.

Lewis-Fernández, R., Balán, I. C., Patel, S. R., Sánchez-Lacay, J. A., Alfonso, C., Gorritz, M., et al. (2013). Impact of motivational pharmacotherapy on treatment retention among depressed Latinos. *Psychiatry, 76*(3), 210–222.

Li, C., Ford, E. S., Zhao, G., Balluz, L. S., Berry, J. T., & Mokdad, A. H. (2010). Undertreatment of mental health problems in adults with diagnosed diabetes and serious psychological distress: The Behavioral Risk Factor Surveillance System, 2007. *Diabetes Care, 33*(5), 1061–1064.

Lin, E. H., Heckbert, S. R., Rutter, C. M., Katon, W. J., Ciechanowski, P., Ludman, E. J., et al. (2009). Depression and increased mortality in diabetes: Unexpected causes of death. *Annals of Family Medicine, 7*(5), 414–421.

Lin, E. H., Katon, W., Von Korf, M., Rutter, C., Simon, G. E., Oliver, M., et al. (2004). Relationship of depression and diabetes self care, medication adherence, and preventive care. *Diabetes Care, 27,* 2154–2160.

Lin, E. H., Rutter, C. M., Katon, W. J., Heckbert, S. R., Ciechanowski, P., Oliver, M. M., et al. (2010). Depression and advanced complications of diabetes: A prospective cohort study. *Diabetes Care, 33*(2), 264–269.

Lin, E. H., Von Korf, M., Ciechanowski, P., Peterson, D., Ludman, E. J., Rutter, C. M., et al. (2012). Treatment adjustment and medication adherence for complex patients with diabetes, heart disease and depression: A randomized control trial. *Annals of Family Medicine, 10*(1), 6–14.

Lundahl, B., & Burke, B. L. (2009). The effectiveness and applicability of motivational interviewing: A practice-friendly review of four meta-analyses. *Journal of Clinical Psychology, 65*(11), 1232–1245.

Lundahl, B. W., Kunz, C., Brownell, C., Tollefson, D., & Burke, B. L. (2010). A meta-analysis of motivational interviewing: Twenty-five years of empirical studies. *Research on Social Work Practice, 20*(2), 137–160.

Madson, M. B., & Campbell, T. C. (2006). Measures of fidelity in motivational enhancement: A systematic review. *Journal of Substance Abuse Treatment, 31,* 67–73.

Madson, M. B., Loignon, A. C., & Lane, C. (2009). Training in motivational interviewing: A systematic review. *Journal of Substance Abuse Treatment, 36,* 101–109.

Magill, M., Apodaca, T. R., Barnett, N. P., & Monti, P. M. (2010). The route to change: Within-session predictors of change plan completion in a motivational interview. *Journal of Substance Abuse Treatment, 38*(3), 299–305.

Maji, D., Shaikh, S., Solanki, D., & Gaurav, K. (2013). Safety of statins. *Indian Journal of Endocrinology and Metabolism, 17*(4), 636–646.

Malerbi, F. E., Negrato, C. A., & Gomes, M. B. (2012). Assessment of psychosocial variables by parents of youth with type 1 diabetes mellitus. *Diabetology Metabolic Syndrome, 4*(1), 48.

Marlatt, G. A., & Donovan, D. M. (Eds.). (2005). *Relapse prevention: Maintenance strategies in the treatment of addictive behaviors* (2nd ed.). New York: Guilford Press.

Martire, L. M., Schulz, R., Helgeson, V. S., Small, B. J., & Saghafi, E. M. (2010). Review and meta-analysis of couple-oriented interventions for chronic illness. *Annals of Behavioral Medicine, 40*(3), 325–342.

Miller, K. M., Beck, R. W., Bergenstal, R. M., Goland, R. S., Haller, M. J., McGill, J. B., et al. (2013). Evidence of a strong association between frequency of self-monitoring of blood glucose and hemoglobin A1c levels in T1D Exchange Clinic Registry participants. *Diabetes Care, 36*(7), 2009–2014.

Miller, W. R. (1983). Motivational interviewing with problem drinkers. *Behavioural Psychotherapy, 11,* 147–172.

Miller, W. R. (1996). What is a relapse?: Fifty ways to leave the wagon. *Addiction, 91*(Suppl.), S15–S27.

Miller, W. R. (2014). Interactive journaling as a clinical tool. *Journal of Mental Health Counseling, 36*(1), 31–42.

Miller, W. R., Forcehimes, A. A., & Zweben, A. (2011). *Treating addiction: A guide for professionals.* New York: Guilford Press.

Miller, W. R., & Moyers, T. B. (2006). Eight stages in learning motivational interviewing. *Journal of Teaching in the Addictions*, 5(1), 3–17.

Miller, W. R., & Muñoz, R. F. (2013). *Controlling your drinking* (2nd ed.). New York: Guilford Press.

Miller, W. R., & Rollnick, S. (1991). *Motivational interviewing: Preparing people to change addictive behavior.* New York: Guilford Press.

Miller, W. R., & Rollnick, S. (2002). *Motivational interviewing: Preparing people for change* (2nd ed.). New York: Guilford Press.

Miller, W. R., & Rollnick, S. (2004). Talking oneself into change: Motivational interviewing, stages of change, and the therapeutic process. *Journal of Cognitive Psychotherapy*, 18, 299–308.

Miller, W. R., & Rollnick, S. (2013). *Motivational interviewing: Helping people change* (3rd ed.). New York: Guilford Press.

Miller, W. R., Yahne, C. E., Moyers, T. B., Martinez, J., & Pirritano, M. (2004). A randomized trial of methods to help clinicians learn motivational interviewing. *Journal of Consulting and Clinical Psychology*, 72, 1050–1062.

Mottillo, S., Filion, K. B., Genest, J., Joseph, L., Pilote, L., Poirier, P., et al. (2010). The metabolic syndrome and cardiovascular risk: A systematic review and meta-analysis. *Journal of the American College of Cardiology*, 56(14), 1113–1132.

Moyers, T. B., & Martin, T. (2006). Therapist influence on client language during motivational interviewing sessions. *Journal of Substance Abuse Treatment*, 30, 245–252.

Moyers, T. B., Martin, T., Catley, D., Harris, K. J., & Ahluwalia, J. S. (2003). Assessing the integrity of motivational interventions: Reliability of the Motivational Interviewing Skills Code. *Behavioural and Cognitive Psychotherapy*, 31, 177–184.

Moyers, T. B., Martin, T., Christopher, P. J., Houck, J. M., Tonigan, J. S., & Amrhein, P. C. (2007). Client language as a mediator of motivational interviewing efficacy: Where is the evidence? *Alcoholism: Clinical and Experimental Research*, 31(Suppl.), 40S–47S.

Moyers, T. B., Martin, T., Houck, J. M., Christopher, P. J., & Tonigan, J. S. (2009). From in-session behaviors to drinking outcomes: A causal chain for motivational interviewing. *Journal of Consulting and Clinical Psychology*, 77(6), 1113–1124.

Moyers, T. B., Miller, W. R., & Hendrickson, S. M. L. (2005). How does motivational interviewing work?: Therapist interpersonal skill predicts client involvement within motivational interviewing sessions. *Journal of Consulting and Clinical Psychology*, 73, 590–598.

Naar-King, S., & Suarez, M. (2011). *Motivational interviewing with adolescents and young adults.* New York: Guilford Press.

National Institute on Alcohol Abuse and Alcoholism. (1996). How to cut down on your drinking. Retrieved from *http://pubs.niaaa.nih.gov/publications/handout.htm.*

National Institute on Drug Abuse. (2010). *Screening for drug use in general medical settings.* Bethesda, MD: National Institutes of Health.

National Institutes of Health. (2011, November 3). What is metabolic syndrome? Retrieved June 29, 2014, from *www.nhlbi.nih.gov/health/health-topics/topics/ms.*

Ogbera, A., & Adeyemi-Doro, A. (2011). Emotional distress is associated with poor self care in type 2 diabetes mellitus. *Journal of Diabetes, 3*(4), 348–352.

Ogedegbe, G., Chaplin, W., Schoenthaler, A., Statman, D., Berger, D., Richardson, T., et al. (2008). A practice-based trial of motivational interviewing and adherence in hypertensive African Americans. *American Journal of Hypertension, 21*(10), 1137–1143.

Pan, X.-R., Li, G.-W., Hu, Y.-H., Wang, J.-X., Yang, W.-Y., An, Z.-X., et al. (1997). Effects of diet and exercise in preventing NIDDM in people with impaired glucose tolerance: The Da Qing IGT and Diabetes Study. *Diabetes Care, 20*(4), 537–544.

Penn, L., White, M., Oldroyd, J., Walker, M., Alberti, K. G., & Mathers, J. C. (2009). Prevention of type 2 diabetes in adults with impaired glucose tolerance: The European Diabetes Prevention RCT in Newcastle upon Tyne, UK. *BMC Public Health, 9,* 342.

Peyrot, M., & Rubin, R. R. (1997). Levels and risks of depression and anxiety symptomatology among diabetic adults. *Diabetes Care, 20*(4), 585–590.

Piette, J. D., Resnicow, K., Choi, H., & Heisler, M. (2013). A diabetes peer support intervention that improved glycemic control: Mediators and moderators of intervention effectiveness. *Chronic Illness, 9*(4), 258–267.

Pouwer, F., Kupper, N., & Adriaanse, M. C. (2010). Does emotional stress cause type 2 diabetes mellitus?: A review from the European Depression in Diabetes (EDID) Research Consortium. *Discovery Medicine, 9*(45), 112–118.

Ratner, R., Goldberg, R., Haffner, S., Marcovina, S., Orchard, T., Fowler, S., et al. (2005). Impact of intensive lifestyle and metformin therapy on cardiovascular disease risk factors in the diabetes prevention program. *Diabetes Care, 28*(4), 888–894.

Resnicow, K., Jackson, A., Braithwaite, R., DiIorio, C., Blisset, D., Rahotep, S., et al. (2002). Healthy body/healthy spirit: A church-based nutrition and physical activity intervention. *Health Education Research, 17*(5), 562–573.

Riley, S. B. (2013). Improving diabetes outcomes by an innovative group visit model: A pilot study. *Journal of the American Association of Nurse Practitioners, 25*(9), 466–472.

Rimm, E. B., Chan, J., Stampfer, M. J., Colditz, G. A., & Willett, W. C. (1995). Prospective study of cigarette smoking, alcohol use, and the risk of diabetes in men. *British Medical Journal, 310,* 555.

Risk Score Profiles. (2013). Framingham Heart Study. Retrieved from *www.framinghamheartstudy.org/risk/coronary.html.*

Roberts, M. (2001). *Horse sense for people.* Toronto: Knopf.

Rogers, C. R. (1959). A theory of therapy, personality, and interpersonal relationships as developed in the client-centered framework. In S. Koch (Ed.), *Psychology: The study of a science: Vol. 3. Formulations of the person and the social contexts* (pp. 184–256). New York: McGraw-Hill.

Rogers, C. R. (1965). *Client-centered therapy.* New York: Houghton Mifflin.

Rogers, C. R. (1980). *A way of being.* Boston: Houghton Mifflin.

Rollnick, S., & Miller, W. R. (1995). What is motivational interviewing? *Behavioural and Cognitive Psychotherapy, 23,* 325–334.

Rollnick, S., Miller, W. R., & Butler, C. C. (2008). *Motivational interviewing in health care: Helping patients change behavior.* New York: Guilford Press.

Rosengren, D. B. (2009). *Building motivational interviewing skills: A practitioner workbook*. New York: Guilford Press.

Rosilio, M., Cotton, J.-B., Wieliczko, M.-C., Gendrault, B., Carel, J.-C., Couvaras, O., et al. (1998). Factors associated with glycemic control: A cross-sectional nationwide study in 2,579 French children with type 1 diabetes. *Diabetes Care, 21*(7), 1146–1153.

Rosland, A. M., Piette, J. D., Choi, H., & Heisler, M. (2011). Family and friend participation in primary care visits of patients with diabetes or heart failure: Patient and physician determinants and experiences. *Medical Care, 49*(1), 37–45.

Rubak, S., Sandbaek, A., Lauritzen, T., & Christensen, B. (2005). Motivational interviewing: A systematic review and meta-analysis. *British Journal of General Practice, 55*, 305–312.

Samuel-Hodge, C. D., Cene, C. W., Corsino, L., Thomas, C., & Svetkey, L. P. (2013). Family diabetes matters: A view from the other side. *Journal of the General Internal Medicine, 28*(3), 428–435.

Scales, R., Lueker, R. D., Atterbom, H. A., Handmaker, N. S., & Jackson, K. A. (1997). Impact of motivational interviewing and skills-based counseling on outcomes in cardiac rehabilitation. *Journal of Cardiopulmonary Rehabilitation, 17*, 328.

Schellenberg, E. S., Dryden, D. M., Vandermeer, B., Ha, C., & Korownyk, C. (2013). Lifestyle interventions for patients with and at risk for type 2 diabetes: A systematic review and meta-analysis. *Annals of Internal Medicine, 159*(8), 543–551.

Shorer, M., David, R., Schoenberg-Taz, M., Levavi-Lavi, I., Phillip, M., & Meyerovitch, J. (2011). Role of parenting style in achieving metabolic control in adolescents with type 1 diabetes. *Diabetes Care, 34*(8), 1735–1737.

Singla, D. R., Weobong, B., Nadkarni, A., Chowdhary, N., Shinde, S., Anand, A., et al. (2014). Improving the scalability of psychological treatments in developing countries: An evaluation of peer-led therapy quality assessment in Goa, India. *Behaviour Research and Therapy, 60*, 53–59.

Smedslund, G., Berg, R. C., Hammerstrøm, K. T., Steiro, A., Leiknes, K. A., Dahl, H. M., et al. (2011). Motivational interviewing for substance abuse. *Cochrane Database of Systematic Reviews* (5), CD008063.

Smith, P. C., Schmidt, S. M., Allensworth-Davies, D., & Saitz, R. (2010). A single-question screening test for drug use in primary care. *Archives of Internal Medicine, 170*(13), 1155–1160.

Sobell, M. B., & Sobell, L. C. (2000). Stepped care as a heuristic approach to the treatment of alcohol problems. *Journal of Consulting and Clinical Psychology, 68*, 573–579.

Stott, N., Rees, M., Rollnick, S., Pill, R., & Hackett, P. (1996). Professional responses to innovation in clinical method: Diabetes care and negotiating skills. *Patient Education and Counseling, 29*, 67–73.

Substance Abuse and Mental Health Services Administration. (2012). *Results from the 2011 National Survey on Drug Use and Health: Summary of national findings* (NSDUH Series H-44, HHS Publication No. [SMA] 12-4713). Rockville, MD: Author.

Svensson, M., Eriksson, J. W., & Dahlquist, G. (2004). Early glycemic control, age at onset, and development of microvascular complications in childhood-onset type 1 diabetes: A population-based study in northern Sweden. *Diabetes Care, 27*(4), 955–962.

Tait, R. J., & Hulse, G. K. (2003). A systematic review of the effectiveness of brief interventions with substance using adolescents by type of drug. *Drug and Alcohol Review, 22,* 337–346.

Tenerz, A., Norhammar, A., Silveira, A., Hamsten, A., Nilsson, G., Ryden, L., et al. (2003). Diabetes, insulin resistance, and metabolic syndrome in patients with acute myocardial infarction without previously known diabetes. *Diabetes Care, 26*(10), 2770–2776.

Tesfaye, S., Boulton, A. J. M., Dyck, P. J., Freeman, R., Horowitz, M., Kempler, P., et al. (2010). Diabetic neuropathies: Update on definitions, diagnostic criteria, estimation of severity, and treatments. *Diabetes Care, 33*(10), 2285–2293.

Tuomilehto, J., Lindstrom, J., Eriksson, J. G., Valle, T. T., Hamalainen, H., Ilanne-Parikka, P., et al. (2001). Prevention of type 2 diabetes mellitus by changes in lifestyle among subjects with impaired glucose tolerance. *New England Journal of Medicne, 344*(18), 1343–1350.

UKPDS Study Group. (1998). Intensive blood-glucose control with sulfonylureas or insulin compared with conventional treatment and risk of complications in patients with type 2 diabetes. *Lancet, 352,* 837–853.

Urbach, S. L., LaFranchi, S., Lambert, L., Lapidus, J. A., Daneman, D., & Becker, T. M. (2005). Predictors of glucose control in children and adolescents with type 1 diabetes mellitus. *Pediatric Diabetes, 6*(2), 69–74.

Vader, A. M., Walters, S. T., Prabhu, G. C., Houck, J. M., & Field, C. A. (2010). The language of motivational interviewing and feedback: Counselor language, client language, and client drinking outcomes. *Psychology of Addictive Behaviors, 24*(2), 190–197.

van Dooren, F. E. P., Nefs, G., Schram, M. T., Verhey, F. R. J., Denollet, J., & Pouwer, F. (Producer). (2013). Depression and risk of mortality in people with diabetes mellitus: A systematic review and meta-analysis. *PLoS One, 8*(3), e57058.

Vanderwood, K. K., Hall, T. O., Harwell, T. S., Butcher, M. K., Helgerson, S. D., & The Montana Cardiovascular Disease and Diabetes Prevention Program Workgroup. (2010). Implementing a state-based cardiovascular disease and diabetes prevention program. *Diabetes Care, 33*(12), 2543–2545.

Vanstone, M., Giacomini, M., Smith, A., Brundisini, F., DeJean, D., Winsor, S. (2013). How diet modification challenges are magnified in vulnerable or marginalized people with diabetes and heart disease: A systematic review and qualitative meta-synthesis. *Ontario Health Technology Assessment Series, 13*(14), 1–40.

Vasilaki, E. I., Hosier, S. G., & Cox, W. M. (2006). The efficacy of motivational interviewing as a brief intervention for excessive drinking: A meta-analytic review. *Alcohol and Alcoholism, 41*(3), 328–335.

Wagner, C. C., & Ingersoll, K. S. (2013). *Motivational interviewing in groups.* New York: Guilford Press.

Weinstein, D. (2014, April 9). Diabetes costliest among non-specialty Rx. Retrieved from *www.mmm-online.com/diabetes-costliest-among-non-specialty-rx/article/342004.*

West, D. S., DiLillo, V., Bursac, Z., Gore, S. A., & Greene, P. G. (2007). Motivational interviewing improves weight loss in women with type 2 diabetes. *Diabetes Care, 30*(5), 1081–1087.

Whittemore, R., Jaser, S., Chao, A., Jang, M., & Grey, M. (2012). Psychological experience of parents of children with type 1 diabetes: A systematic mixed-studies review. *Diabetes Education, 38*(4), 562–579.

Williams, E. D., Rawal, L., Oldenburg, D. F., Renwick, C., Shaw, J. E., & Tapp, R. J. (2012). Risk of cardiovascular and all-cause mortality: impact of impaired health-related functioning and diabetes: The Australian Diabetes, Obesity and Lifestyle (AusDiab) Study. *Diabetes Care, 35*, 1067–1073.

Williams, L. T., Hollis, J. L., Collins, C. E., & Morgan, P. J. (2014). Can a relatively low-intensity intervention by health professionals prevent weight gain in mid-age women?: 12-month outcomes of the 40-something randomised controlled trial. *Nutrition and Diabetes, 4*, e116.

Wood, J. R., Miller, K. M., Maahs, D. M., Beck, R. W., DiMeglio, L. A., Libman, I. M., et al. (2013). Most youth with type 1 diabetes in the T1D Exchange Clinic Registry do not meet American Diabetes Association or International Society for Pediatric and Adolescent Diabetes clinical guidelines. *Diabetes Care, 36*(7), 2035–2037.

Worchel, S. (2013, February 1). Reactance theory. Retrieved from *http://find.gale-group.com/gic/infomark.do?&contentSet=EBKS&idigest=fb720fd31d9036 c1ed2d1f3a0500fcc2&type=retrieve&tabID=T001&prodId=GIC&docId= CX3045302191&source=gale&userGroupName=itsbtrial&version=1.0.*

Xu, Y., Wang, L., He, J., Bi, Y., Li, M., Wang, T., et al. (2013). Prevalence and control of diabetes in Chinese adults. *Journal of the American Medical Association, 310*(9), 948–959.

Index